ACQUIRED
BRAIN INJURY

A Guide for Families and Survivors

Dr Kevin Foy

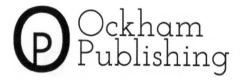
Ockham
Publishing

Figures 1–3, 5, 6, 8, 9: illustrations by Andriy Achyn

Published in 2020 by Ockham Publishing in the United Kingdom

ISBN 978-1-83919-028-5

Cover design by Claire Wood

www.ockham-publishing.com

Dedicated to my patients, colleagues and friends at the Walton Centre with gratitude for everything.

Bridges linking the past and future
old friends passing though with us still.

– Brendan Kennelly, *Begin*

ABOUT THE AUTHOR

Dr Kevin Foy qualified as a doctor from University College Dublin. At an early stage of his training, he developed an interest in the management of patients with acquired brain injury and neuropsychiatric disorders. He trained in psychiatry, obtaining membership of the Royal College of Psychiatrists before spending time training in neurology and obtaining membership of the Royal College of Physicians of Ireland. He completed a Master of Science in Clinical Neuropsychiatry from the University of Birmingham. In 2010, he was awarded a prestigious Doctor Steveen's Scholarship from the Irish Department of Health and spent a year training in the National Hospital for Neurology and Neurosurgery, Queen Square in London. There he worked as a Clinical Fellow in neuropsychiatry and treated patients with diverse neuropsychiatric disease including early onset dementia, Parkinson's disease, Huntington's disease and conversion/psychosomatic disorders.

Since 2011, he has worked as a consultant neuropsychiatrist in Liverpool. Initially he was consultant neuropsychiatrist at the Brain Injury Rehabilitation Centre in Mossley Hill Hospital where he treated individuals with cognitive, behavioural and emotional problems after moderate to severe acquired Brain Injury.

He has also worked at the Walton Centre since 2011 and since 2015 has worked there full time. In the Walton Centre, he assesses and treat patients in tertiary general neuropsychiatry clinics as well as inpatients. He also assesses and manages the inpatients on the three rehabilitation units associated with the Cheshire and Merseyside Rehabilitation and Reablement Network. He has recently started working as a consultant neuropsychiatrist at Bloomfield Health Services, Dublin.

Dr Foy is a national executive committee member of the Faculty of Neuropsychiatry at the Royal College of Psychiatrists. He is the regional specialty representative for neuropsychiatry at the Northern division of the Royal College of Psychiatry. He is also an honorary clinical lecturer at the University of Liverpool and is a visiting lecturer to University of Birmingham.

CONTENTS

INTRODUCTION

Looking back, throughout my childhood and life, I've known countless relatives, neighbours and friends who have suffered an acquired brain injury. At the time, I didn't realise the depth of the struggles and battles they faced on a daily basis. Nobody else seemed to notice either. We all collectively turned a blind eye and looked the other way. We blamed any challenges they had on their idiosyncrasies and disregarded the fact that they had a brain injury.

Acquired brain injury (ABI) is a condition that is far more common in the community than is often realised. Over a million people in the United Kingdom struggle with the long-term consequences of a brain injury. Most of us know individuals who have sustained head injuries or had a brain haemorrhage. Despite this, knowledge about the consequences of the condition is limited among the general public. Even in medical school, I recall little training about ABI. I recall even less in post-graduate training in psychiatry and neurology. In many respects, this is because ABI is, for the most part, a hidden disability and one that doesn't impose upon our consciousness or daily cares. We tend to think erroneously that an individual with a brain injury is somehow fully recovered and back to their old selves when they are discharged from hospital. The day-to-day consequences of acquired brain injury are by and large hidden disabilities, hidden frustrations and hidden sorrows only recognised and experienced by the survivor themselves and their close loved ones.

My own training in relation to the devastating consequences of ABI only really began when I started working as a consultant at both the Merseycare Brain Injury Rehabilitation Unit and at the Walton Centre for Neurology and Neurosurgery in 2011. In both roles, I got the opportunity to learn the complexities of brain injury from my patients and their families.

As a consultant neuropsychiatrist within the Cheshire and Merseyside Rehabilitation Pathway, I have gotten the opportunity to see the journey that an individual and their family makes from the time of the car crash, assault or bleed to their progression within hospital, rehabilitation unit and the community. One of the reasons for writing this book is that the information out there on the internet and in other sources is highly variable; some is frankly incorrect; some is overly optimistic; and some is overly pessimistic.

I hope that this book will give family members and the survivor of ABI a good overview about the condition. I will describe the effects of a brain injury on the brain and body and ultimately how it affects the individual in terms of their memory and cognitive abilities, their mood and their behaviour. I hope this book will also give family members and friends of individuals with a brain injury advice on how to cope with and manage potential challenges in the immediate and longer term.

The first chapters will aim to provide a concise and easy-to-understand overview about the human brain and the various types and severity of brain injuries. Later chapters will look at inpatient care both within the hospital, and rehabilitation units and community care. The physical and mental health consequences of ABI are discussed later in the book, along with specific advice for family members on how to manage such challenges. Throughout the book I'll use illustrative case histories to describe real-world examples of the kind of challenges encountered.

My hope is that survivors and their loved ones can dip in and out of the book and develop a better understanding of the difficulties after a brain injury, and get advice on the potential solutions.

CHAPTER ONE

Welcome to the Brain

In the fourth century B.C., Hippocrates of Cos, the father of medicine, described the brain as the site from which "*arise our pleasures, joy, laughter and jests, as well as our sorrows, pains, griefs and tears*". The human brain is the organ that has led us to walking on the moon and exploring the darkest regions of the universe. The complexity of the brain is awe-inspiring and difficult to contemplate or, for that matter, attempt to summarise in a short chapter. To describe the brain as a computer is to do it a disservice and minimise the complexity of its functions.

THE NEURON IN A NUTSHELL

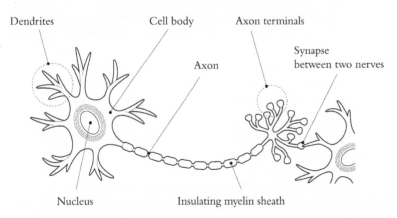

Figure 1: The Neuron

The human brain is essentially a collection of microscopic cells called neurons, with blood vessels and other cells to support them. A neuron is unimaginably small and consists of a headquarters, the nerve cell body and a far smaller cable-like axon that connects it to other nerves and other parts of the body. The nerve cell body can vary in size from 0.004 mm to 0.1 mm – meaning you could fit between one and twenty-five neuron cell bodies side by side across the width of a single human hair. The axon which emerges from the neuron can vary greatly in length, the longest being over three feet long. The diameter of an axon is even smaller at just 0.001 mm or one hundredth the diameter of a human hair. In a similar way that electrical cable is insulated, some axons are covered by a fatty layer called myelin. Myelin functions to speed up the transmission of information through the axon.

Just like people, a neuron is interested in information. The brain can most easily be imagined as being like a very crowded room of people at a party or social gathering. In the case of the brain there are 100 billion neurons and a further ten times that number of cells supporting the individual nerve cells. The supporting cells are called glial cells, and a bit like waiters at a party they support the neurons with nutrients and protection.

Just like party guests, a neuron gets information from many sources – some of which are close in proximity and others which come from further afield such from the foot, hands, eyes, ears, or other sense organs. Whilst each individual guest at a party might have a relatively limited selection of people with whom they communicate, the average neuron has 7,000 connections, also called synapses. And just like a tittle-tattler, the neuron processes such information and sends it to another neuron, or neurons, within microseconds. These other neurons can be located in the brain or the spinal cord. Some people are quite positive and cause other people to laugh or get excited whilst other individuals are negative and depress others – similarly neurons may either be inhibitory and stop other neurons from firing or they can be excitatory and make them fire.

At its most basic, nerve cells communicate with each other through electrical signals. As such, the brain is like an electrical appliance with the electricity flowing along cables – the axons.

The neuron has a different concentration of chemical elements, such as sodium, potassium, and calcium, inside than outside. Just like the ends of a battery, these chemicals all have an electrical charge – either positive or negative. This means that the electrical charge inside the nerve cell is different to that outside. The difference in charge is partly due to pumps within the wall of the neuron that actively pump some chemicals in and others out. Those pumps are switched on or off in response to minute quantities of substances called neurotransmitters which are produced at the end of the axon. The neurotransmitter is secreted into the gap between the neurons and binds to targets on the other neuron causing the pumps in the other neuron to either pump or not pump. The action of the pumps causes the concentration of chemicals and electrical charge within the neuron to suddenly change. Just like a row of dominos falling one by one, the change in the electrical charge moves like a wave down the neuron to the end of the axon, where it stimulates the release of neurotransmitters that cross the gap between neurons and affect the next neuron.

In the same way that at a party, different groups of people will be discussing different things in different parts of the room, different parts of the brain are similarly interested in different functions. Those various parts are linked to each other by the cables of axons that run deep within the brain.

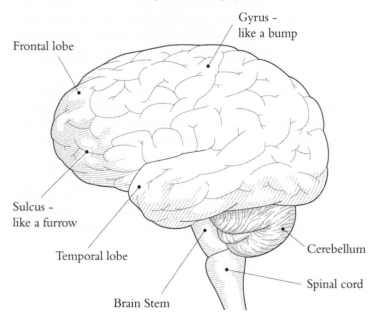

Figure Two: Side View of the Brain

THE BRAIN

The human brain consists of the cerebrum, cerebellum and brain stem. It weighs about 1.5 kg or just over 3 pounds. The cerebrum is the largest part of the brain and is located on the top and in front of the much smaller cerebellum and brain stem. Despite appearing quite solid in photographs or when shown on television documentaries, the cerebrum has the consistency of cold porridge or tofu. It looks a little like a cauliflower with lots of grooves called sulci and elongated bumps called gyri. Scientists and doctors use these grooves and bumps as landmarks when looking at brain scans, completing surgery or when testing how the brain is functioning.

The cerebrum is divided into two halves or hemispheres – one on the left and one on the right. Both hemispheres are connected through a band of tissue called the corpus callosum that lies deep within the brain. Whilst at first glance both hemispheres are mirror images of each other, there are subtle differences particularly in terms of specialised functions. The parts of the brain that have a role in understanding speech and speaking are located on the left in most people. The right side of the brain has an important role in the use of non-verbal information and appears to have a role in taking note of the bigger picture and looking for patterns.

At the back of the brain lies a knob of brain tissue that looks like a miniature brain or a floret of cauliflower glued on. That miniature brain is called the cerebellum and has important roles in controlling movement.

The brain stem is located between the spinal cord and the cerebrum. This part of the brain is vital for the life-supporting systems of the body that control breathing and other essential functions. Damage to this part of the brain is often devastating and causes death.

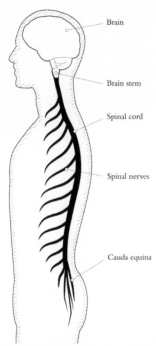

Figure Three: The Spinal Cord

The Cerebrum

As we just introduced, the cerebrum is the main bulk of the brain and sits on top of the brain stem. Each hemisphere is divided into four different lobes which are named after the parts of the skull that cover it: the parietal lobe, the temporal lobe, the occipital lobe and the frontal lobe. Each lobe is associated with performing different functions, and damage to each lobe is associated with differing problems.

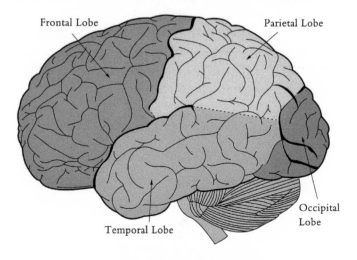

Figure Four: Lobes of the Brain

The temporal lobe is located approximately at the level of the temples and just in front of the ear. It has a number of functions including processing sound information. It also has a role in memory formation. Damage to the temporal lobes can, in some cases, be associated with certain forms of epilepsy.

The parietal lobe sits just above the temporal lobe. This part of the brain receives information from the various sensory organs that are located throughout the body. As a result, this part of the brain processes and integrates information pertaining to touch, pain, temperature of objects and position of parts of the body in space. This information can be used by other regions of the brain, such as the movement centres in the frontal lobe telling a limb to move away from a source of pain.

The parietal lobe also has a role in spatial awareness. Damage of it can lead to sensory neglect meaning that the brain ignores information coming from one part of the body and the individual can end up repeatedly bumping that side of their body.

The occipital lobe is located at the back of the skull. This area receives information from the retina of the eyes and uses the visual information to process and recognise what is in front of the individual. Damage to this part of the brain is associated with different types of blindness.

The Frontal Lobes

The frontal lobes are found at the front of the brain and are especially large in humans, accounting for over 35% of the volume of the whole brain. In comparison, animals have smaller frontal lobes. For example, in dogs the frontal lobe only comprises 7% of the total volume of the brain.

The frontal lobe is divided into the motor cortex, which controls movement, and the pre-frontal cortex, which has important roles in personality, motivation and cognition.

The motor cortex is located towards the back of the frontal lobe and borders the parietal lobe. It makes sense that it is close to the parietal lobe given that movement requires a lot of sensory information. Even though at the level of the naked eye, the strip-like motor cortex all looks the same, its neurons are arranged according to the part of the body they control. Areas of the body that require a lot of precise and delicate movements such as the fingers require far greater control and so have more neurons in the cortex. The areas of the motor cortex that control movement of the mouth and lips is also large given the role the mouth has in communication. The right side of the body is controlled from the left motor cortex and left side is controlled from the right motor cortex. People who write with their right hand are said to have a dominant left hemisphere. Damage to parts of the left motor cortex can profoundly affect speech and the individual's ability to speak. In contrast, damage to the right motor cortex is typically associated with more subtle language changes such as intonation of voice.

The pre-frontal cortex lies in front of the motor cortex. It is the front driving seat of the brain. This part of the brain has very important roles in personality, motivation, social function and cognition. Damage to it can be associated with dramatic changes of personality. This part of the frontal lobe is highly connected with the rest of the brain. As a result, it functions as a supervisor and has an important role in management and organisation. Damage to the frontal lobe is therefore associated with an individual becoming much more disorganised and chaotic – both in terms of their behaviour and also in terms of their ability to memorise things. Through connections with the brainstem, it has an important role in wakefulness. An individual with severe damage to their frontal lobe can present as extremely apathetic and unmotivated.

The frontal lobe is the last part of the brain to develop and fully mature and doesn't stop until the early twenties. Young adults, teenagers and children therefore go around with an immature frontal lobe. This can be readily seen in a school playground or classroom. Younger children can be impulsive in their actions and often take risks without thoughts of the potential consequences. Similarly, they can be blunt in what they say and lack the diplomacy and tact that is supposed to be associated with adulthood. They may also be a little less empathic and sensitive to the needs, desires and feelings of others. Their ability to control their temper can also be less strong than is expected in adults. Similarly, their ability to control their emotions is less robust than in adults – younger children can readily laugh or cry and experience a roller coaster of emotions on a daily basis. All of this is due to the fact that the frontal lobes act as a brake to stop socially inappropriate behaviour. When someone's frontal lobe is damaged, that braking mechanism is affected with quite often significant consequences for how the individual behaves.

The Spinal Cord

The spinal cord descends out of the brain like a long tail. The cord is the thickness of a finger and it starts at the bottom of the skull and is protected by the individual bones of the back which encircle it. The back itself consists of over 24 bones or vertebrae, divided into cervical, thoracic, lumbar, sacral and coccygeal vertebrae. Between the junction of each of the vertebrae, individual string-like nerves emerge out of the spinal cord and break up to supply muscles with information from the brain and carry information back to the brain from sense organs – for example from nerve endings in the skin or joints.

If a telephone cable is cut the message doesn't get through. In a similar way, if the spinal cord is cut, damaged or is starved of blood at any of those various levels information coming from the brain to muscles or to the brain from skin etc. is lost and the person presents with symptoms of paralysis. Complete damage to the spinal cord in the neck is associated with paralysis of all four limbs, also called quadriparesis or tetraparesis. Damage to the spinal cord below the neck is associated with paralysis of the legs.

Blood Supply and the Brain

The brain receives a huge proportion of the blood supply pumped from the heart. Despite the fact that it weighs less than 2% of the total bodyweight, it receives 15% of the blood being pumped from the heart in every beat. Every minute the brain receives the equivalent of 750 mls of blood – that's two and a half soda cans of blood in a minute and 136 cans' worth in an hour. The reason why the blood supply is so high is because the nerve cells within the brain need a lot of oxygen and sugar to keep functioning. Whilst other parts of the body can cope with temporary reductions in blood supply, the brain copes badly with scarcity. Individual nerve cells and parts of the brain are irreparably damaged if there is a loss of blood supply for more than three minutes. One of the parts of the brain which is most sensitive to a lack of oxygen is the hippocampus – the part concerned with taking in information and encoding it to form short-term memory. This is found deep in the temporal lobe. Even quite short periods of loss of blood supply, such as that seen in a cardiac arrest, is enough to irreparably damage this part of the brain causing severe memory problems. The affected individual may be physically quite well after their cardiac arrest and be able to walk and talk but have no ability to recall what is going on in their lives.

As a result of its high requirements for food and oxygen, the brain has a very extensive supply of blood vessels to deliver nutrients and oxygen-rich blood from the heart. The network of blood vessels is more complicated than many other organs of the body and the actual anatomy can vary quite a lot from individual to individual.

PROTECTING THE BRAIN

Bangs to the head are not uncommon. Young children in particular continually fall and play games that risks head trauma. We all have accidentally hit our heads – be it when passing under a low wooden beam or when going up into the loft. This is to say nothing of the knocks to the head when playing football, rugby or other sports. The great miracle of life is why brain injuries aren't more common. Yet if knocks to the head are commonplace now, the frequency of bangs to the head was far more common in history when individuals worked on farms or factories that had little consideration of health and safety. All things considered, humans and other mammals couldn't have been able to evolve without the evolution developing significant protective mechanisms for the brain.

The Skull

The skull, an armour-like protective layer of bone, is a masterpiece of design and engineering. Whilst it is easy to think of the skull as a single bone, it is in fact composed of at least 22 different bones. These bones are fused together, however that fusion doesn't take place until after birth so that the skull can move as it descends through the birth canal when a baby is being born. Within the skull are a number of spaces called sinuses which are air-filled cavities rather than solid bone; the effect of having sinuses means that the head is lighter. Bone itself is incredibly strong – stronger than concrete. The construction of the head itself means that the mid-face and sinuses may act as a kind of crumple zone or relative cushion for protecting the brain.

The Meninges

The brain is protected by three layers that can be compared to bedding on a bed. The innermost layer – similar to a fitted sheet – is called the pia mater (which literally means 'tender mother'). This very delicate and fine spider web-like layer covers the surface of the brain. It is pierced by very small blood vessels called capillaries but otherwise it is impermeable and it seals the brain off and acts like a wax jacket. It has a role in maintaining the blood–brain barrier and isolating the brain from the body so that the nerves within the brain can exist in a delicate environment where chemicals are at a different concentration to the rest of the body.

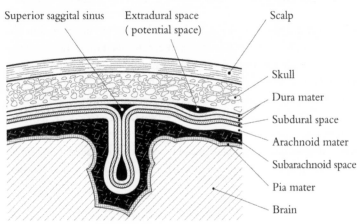

Figure Five: The Meninges

The arachnoid mater is the next layer just above the pia mater. This layer contains the blood vessels, small capillary branches of which divide off and penetrate deeper into the brain. If the pia mater could be considered to be a fitted sheet, the arachnoid mater is best thought of as a bedsheet on top of it. The space between both layers is called the sub-arachnoid layer and is the site where blood collects if a blood vessel bursts, say, as a result of an aneurysm. Normally this layer is bathed in a fine colourless fluid called cerebrospinal fluid.

The outer protective blanket-like layer is called the dura mater, a term derived from Latin and literally meaning 'hard mother'. This layer is very tough and is partly fused to the inside of the skull. Between the dura mater and arachnoid mater is the sub-dural space. This layer contains the bridging veins that can tear in the elderly when the brain shrinks, and produces chronic collections of blood called chronic subdural haemorrhages.

The extradural space lies between the skull and the extradural layer. This contains an artery just around the temple of your forehead that can burst with skull fractures and trauma and bleed causing an extra-dural haemorrhage.

CEREBROSPINAL FLUID AND THE VENTRICULAR SYSTEM

Cerebrospinal fluid (CSF) is a clear fluid that circulates within the brain through a system of cavities and canals called the ventricular system. The brain has around 150 mls, or just under half a lemonade can full of CSF at any one time. However, 500 mls of CSF are produced daily and the fluid circulates and is reabsorbed. There are four ventricles or cavities deep within the brain – two larger lateral ventricles and two smaller ones. The ventricles are connected via small channels and the CSF goes into the subarachnoid space and into a canal in the spinal cord. After some further wandering it is absorbed and passes into the venous system.

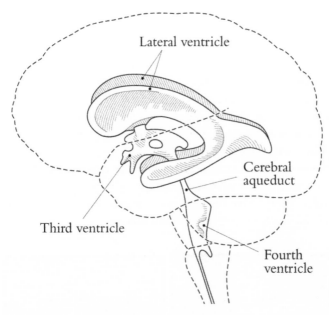

Figure Six: The Ventricular System

CSF and the ventricular system protects the brain in a number of ways. Firstly, it can assist in clearing waste from the brain. Secondly, it can act as a sort of shock absorber. Thirdly, it also functions to support the brain within the closed space of the skull so that the brain almost floats within the fluid.

The protective functions of the CSF system only become problematic if, for a variety of reasons, a blockage develops. This is discussed later in the book in the section describing hydrocephalus.

THE ACHILLES HEEL OF THE BRAIN

The protective system of the brain can also become its worst enemy at times of brain injury. Because the brain lies within a sealed skull, which is in essence like a closed box, problems develop if bleeding occurs within the brain or if the brain itself swells in response to injury. The brain consists of a mixture of brain tissue, blood and cerebrospinal fluid. Any increase in the amount of one of these automatically means a reduction in the amount of space available to the other two. Therefore, if a bleed occurs within the brain, the increased volume of blood leads to increased pressure and this in turn puts pressure on the surrounding brain tissue and CSF volume leading to further brain damage. Similarly, if the brain swells as a result of an infection or in response to damage, this increases the pressure within the skull and runs the risk of reducing blood flow producing further damage. Likewise, blockages within the CSF system lead to a greater volume of CSF and increased pressure and damage to the brain causing reduced blood flow, again, producing further damage. The delicate balance that therefore exists within the brain can be altered as a result of an injury and brain damage begets further brain damage.

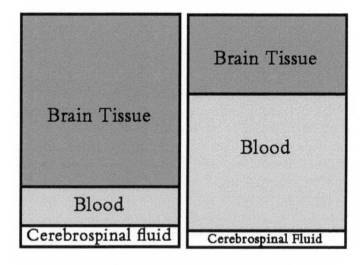

Figure Seven: The delicate balance within the brain: (Left) A normal balance (Right) Effect of bleeding on the brain with increased intracerebral pressure and increased volume of blood.

CHAPTER TWO

What is a Brain Injury?

An acquired brain injury (ABI) is the name given to any damage to the brain that occurs after birth. The damage may be localised to one part of the brain or it may be generalised and affect the whole brain.

When the damage occurs as a result of direct trauma to the brain, such as in a car crash, it is called a traumatic brain injury. ABI may also be the result of a bleed within the brain, lack of oxygen to the brain, an infection or inflammation of the brain, or due to a cancer or an autoimmune process.

TRAUMATIC BRAIN INJURY

Traumatic brain injury occurs as the result of an external force impacting upon the brain, for example, as a result of a fall or assault. That force may be penetrating meaning something actually goes through the skull and directly damages the brain, or be non-penetrating meaning the tough protective skull isn't breached.

Penetrating brain injuries may occur as a result of gunshot wounds to the head or, more commonly in the UK, when an object such as part of a car goes through the skull at speed. In addition to damaging the brain at the point of impact, penetrating brain injuries also introduce potential sources of infection into the brain and as such are very serious. They are associated with far higher rates of subsequent epilepsy than non-penetrating head injuries.

Non-penetrating injuries are just as serious and can occur either due to an object hitting the head, such as occurs in an assault, or due to the rapid acceleration and deceleration forces that occur in a car crash. The brain, as already mentioned, has the consistency of cold porridge and almost floats within the skull thanks to the small layer of cerebrospinal fluid. It is therefore particularly sensitive to sudden forces like when a car hits an object. When this happens, the brain crashes against the inner skull and as it rebounds, the opposite end of the brain hits the inner skull on the other side of the head. This causes what's called a coup and countercoup injury. In addition, rotational forces that cause the brain to twist within the skull at the time of impact are also important. Normally people are facing forward when they are involved in car crashes, so it is the frontal lobe in the front of the brain that gets the immediate impact followed by the back of the brain getting the impact as the brain rebounds.

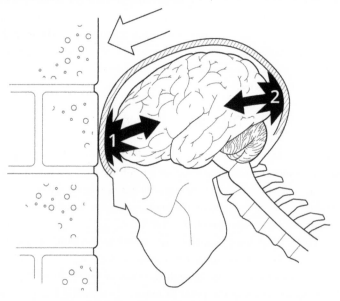

Figure Eight: Coup and Countercoup Injury.

The impact of the brain against the skull can cause some localised bruising and damage to the surface of the brain called a contusion.

Unfortunately, the skull that covers the front part of the brain, especially just behind the eyes, has lots of bony bumps which can grate against and damage the brain underneath after trauma. As we now know, that part of the brain has a particular role in behaviour and in controlling social behaviour and delaying instant gratification. Damage therefore results in significant behavioural issues as we'll see in the chapter on organic personality disorder. The impact of the brain against the skull may also tug on and shear some of the blood vessels in the brain and cause a bleed.

As discussed in chapter 1, the brain consists of billions of individual nerves that are connected by microscopic hair-like wires called axons. In cases where the deceleration forces are particularly strong or cause rotation, the microscopic axons can be cut and sheared apart, or the internal microstructures within may be damaged and cause an injury called diffuse axonal injury. Diffuse axonal injury (DAI) typically occurs deep within the brain. Because the lesions are microscopic, they don't show up well on MRI or CT brain scans and are best seen post-mortem when brain tissue is examined under a microscope. Generally, the presence of DAI can be guessed at through the clinical presentation of the patient and also by the presence of subtle tiny micro-bleeds that may be visible on MRI scanning. Presentations of coma and persistent vegetative states after a brain injury are usually due to DAI. Increasingly, it is believed that some of the symptoms associated with concussion are due to less extensive diffuse axonal injury.

In addition to the direct impact, further brain damage occurs due to chemical changes and the body trying to repair the brain. When nerve cells are damaged, chemicals called neurotransmitters, normally used in small amounts to communicate between nerves, are released in large amounts. Some of these neurotransmitters overexcite other nerves around the damaged area to the extent that those nerves die and release further neurotransmitters. This produces a cascade of more and more death and destruction of neurons – a bit like a set of dominos falling one by one.

The brain is normally protected from various chemicals and toxins within the blood by a blood–brain barrier. This barrier acts like a microscopic raincoat that covers all the blood vessels in the brain meaning that the concentration of chemicals within the brain is very different to that outside the brain. When a piece of brain tissue is damaged, that barrier between the blood vessels and the brain is also damaged. This causes a flood of chemicals from within the blood to leak into the surrounding damaged brain tissue. Some of those chemicals cause further damage and cause the nerve cells to self-destruct. In addition, some of the cells within the brain start to eat up damaged and non-damaged nerve cells and produce more substances that damage cells and cause inflammation.

Inflammation of damaged or injured body tissue is a routine mechanism that the body uses to repair and protect itself. For example, if you hit your thumb accidentally with a hammer, within minutes your thumb will swell up. However, in the enclosed environment of the skull, this works less well. Any swelling within the brain causes pressure to build up in the rest of the brain. That pressure build-up damages more brain tissue, either directly by pushing on it, or indirectly by reducing blood supply to that area of the brain. Occasionally the level of increased pressure can be so high that brain tissue is pushed out or herniates into part of the head causing further brain damage and, frequently, death.

Brain Haemorrhage

A brain haemorrhage is the name given to bleeding that occurs within or around the brain. It damages the brain in two ways: Firstly, through starving the part of the brain that is normally supplied with oxygen and nutrients. Secondly, the additional volume of blood puts pressure on and squashes the surrounding brain tissue. The fact that the brain sits in the skull, which is essentially a closed box, means that any extra blood pooling in the brain as a result of the bleed will displace other brain tissue and damage it.

Brain haemorrhages are a fairly common cause of ABI and many different types exist.

There are many ways of categorising brain haemorrhages but the simplest involves subdividing brain haemorrhages that occur deep within the brain tissue itself, also called intraparenchymal bleeds, and bleeds that occur either under, between, or above the various protective layers of the meninges that cover the surface and outside of the brain.

Intraparenchymal bleeds can occur as a consequence of severe trauma or bangs to the head, burst blood vessels or, rarely, brain tumours. The symptoms that an individual presents with when they have an intraparenchymal bleed is similar to that from other bleeds – namely confusion or suddenly losing consciousness, or sudden loss of functions, such as loss of ability to move a limb, speak, see, or feel things. These bleeds can also occur as a result of uncontrolled high blood pressure.

Intraparenchymal brain haemorrhages are extremely serious and many individuals die either immediately or within weeks of the bleed. Overall nearly half those who suffer a bleed will die within the first month. Those individuals that survive have high levels of disabilities as a result.

Subarachnoid Haemorrhage

As we introduced earlier in chapter one, the brain is protected by three layers called meninges. A bleed that occurs between the middle and deepest layer of the meninges is called a subarachnoid haemorrhage.

Subarachnoid haemorrhages can be caused directly as a result of the brain getting hit or due to spontaneous rupture of the blood vessel. The symptoms of a subarachnoid haemorrhage come on very suddenly, and the resulting headache is described as the worst headache you've ever had. Some doctors refer to it as a "thunderclap headache" as it comes on suddenly and immediately reaches its maximum, just like a clap of thunder. Other symptoms of a subarachnoid haemorrhage include nausea, vomiting or neck stiffness due to irritation of the meninges. However, due to the seriousness of one of these bleeds, the most common symptom is sudden loss of consciousness or becoming confused and drowsy.

Aneurysms

An aneurysm is a localised weakness in the wall of a blood vessel which causes it to bulge. They are a bit like the lump ballooning out of the side of an overly worn car tyre. Aneurysms can develop in blood vessels anywhere within the body, though when they occur in the brain they are associated with certain features. Most are small; however, they can enlarge and produce symptoms due to compressing adjacent nerves. They can be shaped like a berry or can be sausage shaped.

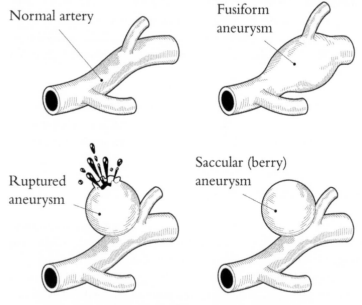

Normal artery

Fusiform aneurysm

Ruptured aneurysm

Saccular (berry) aneurysm

Figure Nine: The Different Forms of Aneurysm

The greatest risk of an aneurysm is that it will burst causing a subarachnoid bleed. Fortunately, most don't – around 3% of the population have asymptomatic aneurysms and the vast majority never rupture. Women seem to be at higher risk of having them than men – twice as likely – and some believe that the reduction of oestrogen after the menopause affects a protein that lines the walls of blood vessels.

Many factors are important in the development of aneurysms. In the vast majority of cases, they are not hereditary and other family members will not develop an aneurysm themselves. Rarely, however, in around 1% of cases, genetic factors are more important and risk is elevated in those families. Screening for undetected aneurysms is available but can have its own problems and the procedure itself isn't risk free. As a result it is generally only recommended for individuals with two or more affected first-degree relatives.

Frequently, aneurysms are incidentally noted when an individual is getting a brain scan for a different reason. If the aneurysm is very small and not causing symptoms, the assessing neurosurgeon will usually decide to monitor the individual and repeat the scan after a period of time (for example six months or a year). They will only decide to intervene if the aneurysm is getting bigger or causing other neurological symptoms. The neurosurgeon may decide to treat the aneurysm by putting a tube into a blood vessel in the groin and threading a very fine wire up through the centre of it and into the brain. The aneurysm can be filled or packed with a fine wire so that the risk of it bursting is reduced. If the aneurysm is bigger or in a difficult position, the neurosurgeon may decide to do more radical treatment by opening the skull and directly treating it. Radiotherapy is also occasionally used to reduce the size of the aneurysm, either on its own or before surgery. All of these interventions are associated with risks, so many individuals with an aneurysm will be monitored rather than given surgery.

Risk of aneurysms is higher in diseases associated with collagen damage such as Marfan's syndrome, polycystic kidney disease, Ehlers Danlos Syndrome and hereditary haemorrhagic telangiectasia. Smoking and untreated high blood pressure are two potentially avoidable risk factors for the development of aneurysms.

Sub-dural Haemorrhage

A further type of bleed that affects the brain is the sub-dural haemorrhage. This can also occur as a result of trauma such as a car accident. However, not infrequently the cause of the trauma can be less obvious and sometimes, especially in the elderly, the trauma can appear to be quite trivial. As we age, our brain shrinks and some of the blood vessels, called bridging veins, between the inside of the skull and brain surface get stretched and put under tension. Fairly minor bangs to the head can cause them to break and bleed. The symptoms of this type of bleed are less dramatic than the subarachnoid haemorrhages. However, nearly half of sufferers lose consciousness immediately. In some individuals, the initial sub-dural bleed may pass unnoticed only for them to become progressively more confused over a number of weeks and eventually lose consciousness or even die. This type of bleed is called a chronic sub-dural haemorrhage.

Extra-dural Bleed

A final type of bleed that is quite rare is called the extra-dural bleed. This typically occurs in younger people and is nearly always associated with skull fractures. The fracture causes an artery close to the inner surface the skull to burst and it bleeds into the space between the skull and the outermost layer of the meninges putting pressure on the brain. The injury is classically associated with sports games and the individual may initially have a period of seeming quite well before becoming more confused and losing consciousness.

(ISCHAEMIC) STROKE

An ischaemic stroke, often just called a stroke, is the second most common cause of death and third most common cause of disability worldwide. Due to the high oxygen requirements of the brain, even a short period of loss of blood supply is enough to cause permanent damage. Ischaemia describes a reduction or cessation of blood supply to a part of the body with resulting damage to body cells. There are three different causes of ischaemic strokes: thrombosis, embolism or reduced blood supply.

Thrombosis occurs when a clot of blood forms inside a blood vessel and blocks it. The body naturally forms blood clots in response to injuries in order to stop bleeding. In strokes due to thrombosis, the clot can be formed due to damaged blood vessel walls. Atherosclerosis

– sometimes called hardening of the arteries – takes place when the inside wall of an artery develops plaques or areas consisting of cholesterol and white blood cells. The cause and development of these plaques is unknown but smoking, diabetes, obesity and high cholesterol appear to be associated with it. There is likely to be a genetic association with development of atherosclerosis and being male also appears to be a risk factor. The atheroma or localised area of atherosclerosis causes the diameter of the blood vessel to progressively get less and less and sometimes the atheroma can burst through the wall of the artery and cause the passing blood to form a clot and block off the vessel. Less commonly, a clot can form as a result of a tear to the wall of the blood vessel, called a dissection. Other less common causes include autoimmune conditions like giant cell arteritis or vasculitis.

An embolism occurs due to a clot or piece of tissue that breaks off and travels in the bloodstream before it blocks an artery that is too small to carry it through. Emboli can develop as a result of physical illnesses elsewhere in the body, and particularly from problems with the heart. Atrial fibrillation – a type of irregular heartbeat – is an important cause of the clots leading to embolism. Other causes of embolism include diseases of the heart muscle, damaged heart valves, or infections of the valves. The symptoms of a stroke due to an embolus are essentially identical to those of thrombosis.

Sudden reduction in blood supply can also cause symptoms of strokes, particularly to areas of the brain that have a poorer supply of blood or to areas of the brain that require a constant source of oxygen and glucose, such as the hippocampus in the temporal lobe. A sudden reduction in blood supply may occur due to cardiac arrest, a large heart attack, a pulmonary embolism (lung clot) or massive blood loss from an accident.

The symptoms of stroke vary widely depending on the part of the brain affected. However, by definition, a stroke is associated with a loss of function of the brain due to blockage of blood supply. If the symptoms last less than 24 hours then they are described as a transient ischaemic attack. If they last longer than 24 hours then it's a stroke.

The classic warning signs of a stroke can be remembered as FAST:

- **Face:** the face droops on one side or an individual may be unable to smile, close their mouth or eyes.
- **Arm:** weakness: being unable to use or raise one's arm, or onset of numbness in a limb or unable to use one's leg.
- **Speech:** being unable to speak or understand what others are saying.
- **Time:** time to call the emergency services.

However, this list of symptoms is quite a simplification and depending on the actual parts of the brain affected, the symptoms experienced can vary greatly between individuals. The key symptom of a stroke is its sudden onset of loss of function or altered function. Strokes in the back of the brain can be associated with the onset of nausea, dizziness, double vision, numbness of the face, or sudden clumsiness of a limb or onset of numbness or difficulty swallowing. Strokes of blood vessels in the front of the brain can cause speech problems, arm or leg weakness, problems with spatial awareness, blindness or loss of parts of vision. Strokes to some parts of the brain can appear silent and aren't associated with dramatic changes, although they are associated with subtle changes in cognition and sometimes confusion.

The most important thing about a stroke is the sooner an individual attends hospital, the better. A stroke is usually diagnosed through a history and physical examination but will be confirmed through brain scans such as a CT brain or MRI. Prompt diagnosis may enable the use of clot-busting drugs to dissolve the stroke and reduce the level of permanent damage and disability.

Cerebral Venous Thrombosis

A cerebral venous sinus thrombosis (CVT) is a very rare form of stroke that occurs when a blockage forms in the large channels that exist between the layers of the outermost meninges – the dura into which the veins of the brain drain into. These sinuses eventually drain into the internal jugular vein that goes into the neck and eventually the heart.

Cerebral venous thrombosis is more difficult to diagnose than other strokes and presents with a number of different symptoms that can be often quite vague. Individuals that are affected by these strokes are younger and are most commonly women. Being pregnant and the period after delivery of the baby are associated with higher risks of its development. Other causes can include clotting disorders, cancer and a number of chronic inflammatory conditions.

The most common symptom seen in CVT is headache – it often develops gradually over a number of days but can be quite variable and difficult to distinguish from a migraine in some.

SUMMARY

The causes of ABI are many and can include both traumatic brain injury and bleeds. However, no acquired brain injury is the same and many, particularly individuals who've sustained a traumatic brain injury, will develop brain damage due to a combination factors including bruising, bleeds, diffuse axonal injury and lack of oxygen.

CHAPTER THREE

Acquired Brain Injury: The Silent Epidemic

It comes as a shock to many people that ABI is a major cause of both death and disability in the world. A total of 9% of world deaths and 12% of chronic ill health is due to brain injury. In addition, ABI is a major cause of death in the under 40s. Rates of acquired brain injury – particularly traumatic brain injury – is rising throughout the world, especially in developing nations due to more cars being on the road. The actual incidence of traumatic brain injury varies greatly between each country and is influenced greatly by factors such as the percentage of young adults (particularly young males) in the population, road infrastructure, road traffic speed laws and enforcement, and access to guns.

There are many reasons for why acquired brain injury is a hidden disability. However, one of the major reasons is due to poor collection of data. In the UK, most data in casualty departments is coded by extremely junior administration staff who have a tendency to give priority to more overt problems such as fractured arms or legs, than notice any associated secondary head injuries. Indeed, it is estimated that less than 50% of data is coded correctly. Other causes of ABI, such as brain haemorrhages and infections, are coded even worse. Unfortunately, the nature of the NHS means that the absence of joined-up thinking and joined-up following of patients means that the data itself is highly inaccurate. One study suggests that brain injury could be up to six times higher than actually reported.[1]

What we do know is that brain injury is extremely common. In the UK alone, 1.4 million people attend hospital with traumatic brain injuries annually.[2] In terms of severity, nearly 90% of people with a traumatic head injury are discharged within 24 hours. Of those with more severe acquired brain injuries, up to one-third will suffer some degree of medical complication; more often that of pneumonia, as well as sepsis and other physical problems.

The period 2016-2017 saw over 340,000 people admitted with some degree of brain injury problems in the UK; 156,000 of those were directly due to traumatic brain injury; and 132,000 were due to strokes.[3] Brain injury is at least 1.5 times more common in men than women, although the rates of brain injury in women over a ten-year period have increased by up to 24%.

The rates of brain injury are higher in young people and in the very elderly. The causes of brain injury in the elderly are usually falls or strokes. In younger people, the causes are road traffic accidents and assaults.

A number of other factors associated with brain injury include poverty, urban living and deprivation. Similarly, alcoholism and drug use are also associated with higher rates of brain injuries. In the United States gun crime and suicide attempts through the use of firearms is a major cause of traumatic brain injury.

---

[1] Incidence of traumatic brain injury in New Zealand: a population-based study, V Feigin et al, Lancet Neurology 2013

[2] National Institute for Health and Clinical Excellence: Guidance. Head injury: triage, assessment, investigation and early management of head injury in children, young people and adults. London: National Institute for Health and Care Excellence (UK), 2014

[3] Headway: The Brain Injury Association

COSTS TO SOCIETY

Despite being considered a hidden disability, there is evidence of the consequences of brain injury everywhere. The costs of ABI are enormous, with costs of traumatic brain injury alone in the United States estimated to be $76.5 billion, and stroke $54 billion per annum in 2010 based on a 2001 study.[4] The costs of traumatic brain injury in the United Kingdom are less well known, but were estimated in 2010 to be somewhere between £4.1 billion and £15 billion.[5] At least one million individuals live with the long-term consequences of acquired brain injury in the United Kingdom. These individuals have higher social care costs and health costs than the general population, therefore, the annualised cost of brain injury is likely to be an underestimate.

SOCIAL OUTCOME AFTER A BRAIN INJURY

Statistics in terms of the percentage of people with moderate to severe brain injury who return to work are highly variable. Less than 50% of survivors will be working two years after their injury, and if someone does not return to work within these two years, they are highly unlikely to ever return to work.[6]

In the past, it was believed that rates of divorce were far higher in those who suffered a brain injury than those who did not. A number of studies from the 1980s conducted in the United States suggested that between 48% and 78% of people ended up getting up divorced after a brain injury. However, more recent studies have tended to suggest that rates of divorce are far lower. At least 75% of people remain

---

[4] E. Finkelstein, P. Corso, T. Miller et al., The Incidence and Economic Burden of Injuries in the United States. New York (NY): Oxford University Press; 2006
[5] M. Parsonage. Traumatic brain injury and offending: an economic analysis. July 2016 Centre for Mental Health
[6] J. Dudok, et al. How many people return to work after acquired brain injury: a systematic review. Brain Injury, (2009) 23(6) 473-88

married after a brain injury, although rates of divorce do appear to be higher in males who have a brain injury than in females.[7]

At first glance, homelessness would appear to be a disturbing consequence of brain injury. A recent study that looked at well-designed studies from six high-income countries found that over half of homeless people had previously suffered a brain injury. These brain injuries were often severe and a quarter of the homeless population's studies had moderate to severe brain injuries.[8] Closer to home, a similar small study from Leeds in 2010 found that 48% of the homeless population there had a history of brain injury.[9] That said, the causes of ABI are many, as indeed are the causes of homelessness, and it is highly likely that factors common to both homelessness and ABI, such as alcoholism, drug use and co-morbid mental illness, may also be the cause of the apparent association between the two.

A similar confounding association is likely to be between rates of acquired brain injury in the prison populations. A recent study found that 60% of UK prisoners self-reported a history of brain injury. Prisoners who've sustained a brain injury offend at an earlier age, reoffend more, get longer sentences and are seven times more likely to have co-morbid mental illness.[10]

In addition, at least 50% of people in long-term medium to secure forensic units have problems associated with acquired brain injury.

---

[7] J Kreutzer, the truth about divorce after traumatic brain injury Brainline.org

[8] J Stubbs et al. Traumatic brain injury in homeless and marginally housed inmdividuals: a systematic review and meta-analysis. The Lancet Public Health Dec 2019

[9] Disabilities Foundation 2010

[10] W Huw Williams Traumatic brain injury: a potential cause of violent crime. *Lancet Psychiatry* 2018 5(10) 836-44

SUMMARY

Acquired brain injury is anything but an uncommon problem. Whilst only a minority of people offend or become homeless after a brain injury, prison and homeless shelter populations have a disproportionate history of ABI. It is a hidden disability due to a number of factors; most notably inadequate statistics and a tendency of both government and society as a whole to look the other way.

CHAPTER FOUR

Mild, Moderate or Severe?

Determining outcome after a brain injury is a challenge at the best of times. Patience and the passage of time are ultimately the best at determining prognosis in the longer term. The most important factor in determining outcome after a brain injury is the severity of the initial brain trauma itself. The simple fact is people with bad head injuries do worse. Clinicians routinely categorise brain injuries into three categories: mild, moderate and severe. The criteria used to determine severity varies from country to country but most use three factors: Glasgow Coma Scale (GCS), period of loss of consciousness and period of confusion after regaining consciousness – the so-called PTA (post-traumatic amnesia) duration.

GLASGOW COMA SCALE

GCS is used to determine the level of consciousness using a number of simple neurological tests that can be performed at the scene of the accident by paramedic staff, and during inpatient stay. These tests include how responsive the patient is – whether they respond to various stimuli such as noise or pain; whether they can obey a simple command; whether they can open their eyes; and whether they can talk or if their speech is comprehensible. The patient's best motor, verbal and eye-opening responses are noted and assigned a numerical grade. The three responses add up to a maximum of 15. The GCS score for being completely conscious and alert is therefore 15. Those who are alert but confused get a total of 14. The lowest score possible – seen

31

in those who are profoundly unconscious or brain dead – is 3. By definition, GCS in mild brain injury is between 13 and 15. In moderate brain injury it is between 9 and 12 and those with severe brain injury have a GCS of less than 8.

LOSS OF CONSCIOUSNESS

Even though loss of consciousness is a well-known immediate consequence of ABI, the actual cause of what happens at a brain or cellular level to cause people to lose consciousness remains a bit of a mystery with a number of different theories. What is known is that the duration of loss of consciousness is reflective of the severity of the brain damage. Those with more minor head injuries will either not lose consciousness or be knocked out for less than 30 minutes. Those with a moderate head injury will have loss of consciousness for more than 30 minutes but less than 24 hours. Loss of consciousness for more than 24 hours is associated with a severe head injury.

POST-TRAUMATIC AMNESIA

Post-traumatic amnesia (PTA) is the duration of confusion after regaining consciousness when an individual is unable to register new memories and is generally disorientated in time and place. This period will be described in greater detail in chapter 13. Those with a mild brain injury will have confusion on regaining consciousness for less than 24 hours. Those with moderate brain injuries will have PTA duration of more than 1 day but less than 7 days. Those affected with the more severe brain injuries will have a PTA of more than a week.

THE MYTH OF MILD BRAIN INJURY?

Despite its name, there is nothing necessarily mild about a 'mild brain injury'. A number of studies have found that very subtle abnormalities such as micro haemorrhages may be seen on the brain scans of people who fulfil the criteria for mild brain injury. Individuals with a mild brain injury will also usually experience physical, cognitive and emotional symptoms afterwards – though for the most part these symptoms are self-limiting. Further information is mentioned in chapter 14.

OUTCOME IN MORE SEVERE BRAIN INJURIES

The outcome for those with moderate and severe brain injuries is less positive and both are associated with longer hospitalisations, more disability and challenges with cognition, memory and behaviour. Since brain injuries by their nature are all very different, despite a severe injury some people can have surprisingly positive outcomes in terms of ability to live and function independently. The factors associated with outcome include age (those with advanced age generally do poorer), pre-injury medical, psychiatric or substance misuse problems, and the development of medical complications post-injury such as increased intracranial pressure or hydrocephalus. The location of the injury itself is also an important outcome factor with frontal lobe injuries being associated with more behavioural challenges, which we'll look at more in chapter 12.

CHAPTER FIVE

Investigations and Tests

Development of technology has revolutionised the management and care of individuals after brain injuries. It is still within living memory that the only type of X-ray that could be used for looking at the brain was a simple skull X-ray. The recent development and widespread availability of CT and MRI scanners has revolutionised how we can investigate and diagnose brain injuries.

CT AND MRI SCANS

Computerised tomography scans, or CT or CAT scans, are a special form of X-ray that can produce images of what various parts of the body would look like in a sliced format – a bit like looking at the individual slices in a loaf of bread. In the case of the brain they can show what the brain tissue inside the brain looks like. They are best at showing areas of bleeding and broken bone but sometimes dye can be injected to highlight particular blood vessels in the brain. The great advantage of CT scans is that they can be performed fairly quickly.

Magnetic resonance imaging, (MRI) or MR scans, can also produce images of what the inside of the brain looks like. Again, they can show slices of what the brain looks like but unlike CT Brains, the scans can be altered to highlight different abnormalities or look at different brain tissue. They show black-and-white images of the brain that are remarkably vivid and clear, and improved technology means that they are even more sensitive at detecting changes within the brain. Again, similar to CT scans, intravenous substances can be injected to highlight particular areas of blood vessels, particularly in cases of aneurysms or vascular changes in the brain. The MRI uses very powerful magnets and even more powerful computers to produce the image. On a practical level, because magnets are used, individuals who have old metal implants such as certain types of heart valves or bone replacements might not be able to utilise MRI scanners. A bigger problem lies in the fact that MR scanning is slower than CT scans and the machine makes a lot of noise in the process. An individual having the scan will have to lie very still for up to 30 minutes and this can be a problem, especially in individuals with confusion or claustrophobia.

ECG

Electroencephalography, or EEG, is used to examine electrical brain waves. The nerves within the brain use electrical energy in the transmission of information and very sensitive equipment can be used to look at the pattern of the electrical output from various parts of the brain. This can be useful in determining whether the brain is still working and can be used to declare brain death in intensive care situations. It can also be useful in the diagnosis of epilepsy and is sometimes used when an individual is very confused.

LUMBAR PUNCTURE

Lumbar puncture is an investigation rarely used in brain injury but can be used to diagnose infections within the brain like encephalitis or meningitis. As mentioned earlier, the brain contains up to 150 mls of cerebrospinal fluid in ventricles going down the spinal canal and into the spinal cord. Thanks to the oddities of human anatomy, it is possible to get a sample of this fluid by inserting a long and fine needle between bones at a place in the lower back where nerves of the spinal cord float. Obtaining fluid can be a challenge especially in those who are very confused and unable to bend their back in such a way to allow the needle to get in between the bones. Very little fluid is removed but it can be tested for amounts of protein, blood cells and bacteria as well as other chemicals to help diagnose serious infections within the brain.

BLOOD TESTS

It is very difficult to be admitted to any hospital without having blood tests. Blood tests in the context of brain injury are generally to rule out other medical problems that can occur in the context of trauma and also to monitor how well other organs, such as the kidneys and liver, are working. At present, there isn't a blood test used in routine clinical practice to determine the severity of a brain injury. A number of blood tests to detect concussion are being investigated and developed, however they have yet to enter routine clinical practice and at this stage are only being used in research settings.

CHAPTER SIX

Neurosurgery and Initial Inpatient Care

The vast majority of acquired brain injuries are managed at local district general hospitals. Over 80% of traumatic brain injuries are defined as being mild and most are discharged home from casualty the same day.

Most individuals with moderate to severe traumatic brain injuries will be treated at their local district general hospital. This is entirely appropriate in the vast majority of cases. However, individuals who show evidence of more severe brain injury and, in particular those who have significant abnormalities on their CT or MRI brain scans, may be seen by neurosurgeons at the regional neuroscience or neurotrauma centres. Patients will only be transferred to these centres if there is evidence of brain damage that requires either neurosurgical monitoring or neurosurgical intervention itself.

Even for those individuals who are transferred to the regional neuroscience centre, most will not have an operation or surgical intervention. Instead, the neurosurgeon and their team will closely monitor the patient and monitor their scans. The patients may be treated in intensive care or high-dependency units or, indeed, on a general surgical ward.

Clotted blood may occasionally accumulate in the brain as a result of the brain trauma or bleed. The neurosurgeons will only manage this and intervene with surgery if the clot is so large that it is putting pressure on the brain.

In cases of chronic subdural haematomas, a small hole can be drilled into the skull and the blood clot, which in this circumstance can be quite liquid-like, can be drained.

In cases where fresher or hard clotted material is putting pressure on the brain, the neurosurgeon may have to perform an operation called a craniotomy. The individual will be taken to theatre and part of the skull is drilled open to allow removal of the clot.

A somewhat simpler procedure is intracranial pressure monitoring (ICP). This is a procedure which is used if the neurosurgeons are concerned that there is a risk of raised intracranial pressure. Raised intracranial pressure is a very serious complication of a brain injury and occurs when the brain tissue swells inside the skull. As already mentioned, due to the fact that there is little room for expansion of the skull, this can lead to further brain damage. ICP is performed using a very simple wire which is connected to a machine and can monitor the pressure within the skull.

Raised intracranial pressure is most normally treated by sedating the patient and giving them intravenous fluids and other medication to lower pressure. Occasionally, in some settings, the patient might get extra oxygen to try and reduce the swelling.

However, sometimes simple monitoring and treatment in an induced coma is not sufficient. In those cases, the brain can become potentially very swollen and lead to further brain damage. When this happens, neurosurgeons will take the patient to theatre and remove a section of the skull, leaving it off for weeks or even months. This procedure is called a decompressive craniectomy. It allows the brain to expand without damaging it further. The brain itself is covered over with skin and the patient is returned to intensive care. At a later date, the skull can be replaced or a special plastic patch can be reconstructed to cover the area where the skull was removed. This type of operation is called a cranioplasty. Neurosurgeons delay offering a cranioplasty until firstly, the swelling has settled and, secondly, they have made sure that there is no risk of infection.

One of the other potential complications of a brain injury is hydrocephalus, which is a collection of too much cerebrospinal fluid

(CSF) due to a blockage of the ventricular system with resulting raised pressure on the surrounding brain tissue. Hydrocephalus can produce symptoms of headaches, confusion, nausea, unsteadiness and a number of other neurological signs. Untreated, hydrocephalus can be fatal. Neurosurgeons will manage it by inserting a small tube, an external ventricular drain, to drain away the extra CSF.

LIBERTY PROTECTION SAFEGUARDS (FORMERLY DoLS)

Once upon a time, not so long ago, any individual who was vulnerable and needed to be in hospital was kept in hospital. If they were confused and wanted to leave, they were made to remain against their will. They weren't sectioned under the mental health act. There was no additional paperwork required and they were kept under 'common law' because it was felt it would be unwise and irresponsible to let them out of the hospital. The enactment of the Human Rights Act (1998) in the UK meant that holding any individual on a hospital ward against their will (even if they needed to be there) was deemed to be illegal. In England and Wales, the Mental Capacity Act and in particular the deprivation of liberty safeguards was enacted to plug that gap and to allow clinicians keep patients who were clearly vulnerable and needed care in hospital and other care related facilities.

As from October 2020, any patient who lacks capacity will be detained in hospital against their will using the Liberty Protection Safeguards (LPS) in England and Wales. Prior to that changeover, the Deprivation of Liberty Safeguards (DoLS) is in use. To place someone on LPS or DoLS the treating team need to be of the opinion that the individual needs to be in hospital but lacks the capacity to make that decision themselves.

To be considered to lack capacity, an individual has to have a disorder of brain or mind, such as an episode of confusion after a brain injury. As a result of that disorder, the individual should have difficulties with either understanding or recalling information or with using that information to come to a reasoned, well-thought-out decision. If the individual also has a severe communication problem to the extent that meaningful communication is impossible, they are also considered to lack capacity. One of the hallmarks of the Mental Capacity Act is that everyone is deemed to have capacity until proven otherwise and individuals are all allowed to make unwise decisions if they are deemed to have capacity.

As part of being placed on LPS, if the individual objects and still wants to leave, the hospital will arrange for them to be assessed by an Approved Mental Capacity Professional, usually a social worker.

Being on LPS is different to being sectioned under the Mental Health Act. Use of the Mental Health Act in acquired brain injury is relatively uncommon and isn't used in the acute setting.

The other constituent nations of the United Kingdom have different versions of LPS but the principles of capacity remain the same. Despite plans to introduce a version of deprivation of liberty in the Republic of Ireland – called the assisted decision making – the legislation has been passed by Dáil Éireann hasn't been enacted yet and use of 'common law' detentions remain.

CHAPTER SEVEN

Rehabilitation: A Multidisciplinary Journey

After the initial inpatient treatment phase is completed, the next stage of treatment is rehabilitation. Rehabilitation is the name given to the work performed which aims to maximise the abilities of the individual. It is collaborative, meaning that the patient is very much a partner in their rehabilitation and needs to actively work with therapists in planning goals. It is also multidisciplinary meaning that a number of different specialists from different therapies work together as part of the rehabilitation team. Rehabilitation starts very early and for some will start when the individual is still in intensive care with physiotherapists working to prevent development of problems such as spasticity or chest infections. The therapies are offered in a number of settings from intensive care units, to general hospital wards, to specialist rehabilitation units and ultimately to the community. The duration of rehabilitation varies; those with severe behavioural or medical problems may not be ready for rehabilitation straight after their injury and so may end up going to other facilities before they are emotionally and physically ready for the arduous and active task of rehabilitation.

A number of professionals work within rehabilitation and it can be rather confusing understanding what the roles of the various therapists are.

REHABILITATION CONSULTANT

A rehabilitation consultant is a medical doctor with specialist training in rehabilitation medicine. They are interested in the assessment and management of difficulties encountered as a consequence of brain injury and will treat day-to-day medical problems for the duration of inpatient rehabilitation. Problems can include common medical issues such as chest and urinary tract infections and problems with pain. They also have a special role in the management of complications such as spasticity when a limb becomes fixed and difficult to move due to nerve damage. Rehabilitation doctors will have a particular role in the management of prosthetics for individuals who have limbs amputated as a result of trauma.

The speciality originally developed as a consequence of the First World War where a large number of former soldiers were left with severe physical deficits such as loss of limbs.

PHYSIOTHERAPISTS

Physiotherapists are qualified health professionals and have a number of roles within rehabilitation. They will assist the patient with exercises to help breathing and reduce the risks of phlegm collecting in the lungs – this is particularly important when the patient is in intensive care or recovering from surgery. They also help to prevent development of spasticity in the limbs and will regularly visit the individual and do exercises with limb movement. In the early phase of rehabilitation the individual may have problems with feeling dizzy if they have to sit up, and their body may weaken to the point that it is unable to sustain their bodyweight. The physiotherapist will use a piece of equipment called a tilt table to help the individual become used to being upright again. The equipment itself looks like a medieval torture instrument but is essentially a table with belts to hold the patient in place whilst it is gradually moved from being flat to upright. Over time the individual will be able to tolerate being upright as their strength improves. When the patient is able to be upright for longer periods, the physiotherapists will then start getting them back standing again and train them in the use of walking aids and crutches. Prior to discharge, the physiotherapist will have a role in the assessment of whether the individual is safe in terms of mobilising at home and they will work along with occupational therapy in terms of whether any additional aids are required.

OCCUPATIONAL THERAPISTS

Occupational therapists, or OTs, are qualified professionals whose role is to work with the individual and make them as independent as they safely can be in day-to-day life. They will help with the management of any confusion and will use charts and notices to try and remind the individual where they are and what has happened to them. As the individual gets better, they assess the ability of the individual to complete everyday tasks such as getting dressed, showering, and participating at mealtimes. A specially adapted OT kitchen is used to assess safety within the kitchen environment. Patients with brain injuries and their relatives are frequently confused as to why so much care is placed into assessing safety within the kitchen. This is generally because the kitchen contains equipment that can cause injury and it is a good way of assessing how safe they are in other parts of the home. OTs also have an important role in assessing the skills an individual will have off the ward and in public spaces. They will frequently assess the individual's ability to safely cross roads and do daily tasks such as going to a shop. Prior to discharge, they will assess the individual's ability to manage in their own home and will advise family on additional adaptations to the home that might be needed.

SPEECH THERAPISTS

Speech and language therapists, often abbreviated to SLTs, are professionals whose expertise lies in communication. In the context of brain injury, they assess the individual's ability to safely swallow food and drink fluids. Those with impaired swallow are at a high risk of getting serious lung infections due to aspiration. The SLT will assess this and may advise staff to alter the individual's diet and add substances to thicken the fluids so that they can be swallowed more safely. Their other role lies in the assessment or treatment of communication diffi-culties. When they assess communication, they will be interested in both verbal and non-verbal communication. In terms of verbal, they will assess the individual's ability to understand what others say as well as the ability to speak themselves. In cases where the individual has difficulty speaking, the SLT will work with them breaking up speech and doing various exercises. For those with more serious speech and communication problems the SLT can aid communication through the use of technology.

DIETICIAN

Serious brain injuries are associated with loss of weight in the acute phase of treatment. This happens for a number of reasons: Firstly, when a body is injured it requires more energy to repair tissue. Sec-ondly, in the immediate aftermath of an injury the individual may be unconscious and therefore unable to eat. Thirdly, swallowing issues may interfere with the ability to consume as much food as they nor-mally would. The rate of weight loss can vary depending on these and a number of other factors. As a result, nursing staff closely monitor weight and body mass index and how much the patient is eating. Damage to certain organs can mean that the patient will be unable to process, or will be deficient in, certain nutrients. The dietician will work closely with medical and nursing staff in these situations and will prescribe diets and additional foods and supplements for the patient to optimise their weight.

PSYCHOLOGISTS

Psychologists are highly skilled professionals whose area of expertise lies in identification and management of cognitive and emotional problems. In the context of brain injury, psychologists will have par-ticular expertise in the assessment of cognitive problems through use of neuropsychological tests. Such tests can identify which parts of the brain aren't functioning well. These tests can also estimate the level of changes due to the brain injury and can also compare the individual's ability with that of the general population. MRI and CT scans currently have only limited abilities to define the memory and other learning problems after a brain injury. Psychologists, however, can identify which parts of the brain are damaged and potentially measure the recovery over time. This can greatly assist other members of the rehabilitation team.

The whole process of rehabilitation can be very stressful and psychologists offer techniques to manage distress. These talking therapies include counselling, cognitive behavioural therapy (CBT) and mindfulness, and sometimes group work. As such the psychologist can have a very close and personal role to play with the survivor during the journey of recovery. Psychologists also offer support to family members who may be distressed and overwhelmed by the emotions in the aftermath of a brain injury.

A neuropsychologist is a psychologist with special expertise on the effect of ABI and other physical conditions of the brain on behaviour, thinking and feelings.

SOCIAL WORKERS

Social workers have a particular area of expertise in liaising with agencies and planning and co-ordinating discharge packages of care. In the case of complex disabilities, the additional supports required to facilitate a safe discharge can involve several government and private agencies. Discharge preparation is even more complex if the individual experienced social difficulties before the injury such as substance misuse, accommodation issues or if the patient has parental responsibilities. Getting funding for such packages is complex and increasingly complicated. The social worker has to run the gamut of getting funding whilst organising the package and at the same time being mindful of the finite nature of funds available for support. On discharge the social worker will have a role in following the individual up and in managing any additional issues that will invariably arise when they are discharged.

NURSING

The professional at the coalface of rehabilitation is the nurse. On a day-to-day basis they manage the patient and look after their physical, psychological and social needs whilst managing any behavioural difficulties at the same time. In the case of brain injury they have a particular role in preventing the many consequences of prolonged immobility and bed rest, such as bed sores. They monitor the patient for the development of any new onset medical problems such as urinary tract infections or pneumonias, which can develop suddenly and can be life threatening in the physically vulnerable state after an accident. They dispense medications and look for any side effects of medications. They assist with the activities of daily living such as getting up, getting dressed, eating, washing and going back to bed. Whilst other specialists have a role in offering therapy to the patient, the nurse is the professional who implements the actual treatments. The nurse is the one who has to deal with and manage behavioural problems whilst at the same time being cognisant of the other patients on the ward and their needs. A rehabilitation nurse invariably has skills in a number of areas, particularly in the arts of encouragement and cajoling patients with confusion or agitation. Prior to discharge they also have a role in liaising with staff in care facilities or with district nursing.

NEUROPSYCHIATRISTS

Neuropsychiatrists are first and foremost medical doctors. They have a particular interest in conditions that span between psychiatry and neurology and as such cover the grey area between brain and mind. In the case of ABI, they will assess cognition and behaviour and look for any associated psychiatric problems such as depression or anxiety. Individuals who suffer a brain injury not infrequently have problems with mental health and substance misuse that predates the injury. In the busy rehabilitation environment, such difficulties may be missed so the neuropsychiatrist has a role in the identification of mental health problems during rehabilitation. Agitation and behavioural problems are common after a brain injury; the neuropsychiatrist manages such difficulties using both non-medical and medical interventions. In terms of longer-term planning, the neuropsychiatrist has a role in advising of the optimal placement on where the individual should reside, both for the individual's safety and the safety of others. They follow up and manage longer-term difficulties of agitation, anger problems and frontal lobe personality problems.

There are a small number of medications that can help with memory problems; the neuropsychiatrist will have the particular knowledge in the use of these tablets. They will frequently assess the capacity of the individual and give an opinion as to the degree of insight the individual has in relation to their cognitive problems and any associated risks. Rehabilitation units that specialise in behavioural problems are usually run by neuropsychiatrists who work alongside members of the multidisciplinary team in the management of behavioural problems after a brain injury.

CHAPTER EIGHT

Inpatient rehabilitation

REHABILITATION SETTINGS

Rehabilitation units throughout the country, and the world, vary quite a lot with the care they provide. Some units treat patients at different stages of their recovery, or specialise in management of different conditions after brain injury (such as low awareness states or resulting mental health problems) whereas others offer more generalised treatment. Some units offer shorter-term rehabilitation whilst others offer longer-term rehabilitation. Increasingly, many units are run by the private sector, particularly those treating longer-term behavioural problems such as organic personality disorder post brain injury. The NHS rehabilitation units treat individuals for shorter periods of time. They are frequently located on the site of regional neuroscience or trauma centres but can also be stand-alone units. The benefits of being located on the site of a neuroscience unit is that patients have access to support from clinicians within that centre in the event of any complications or problems developing.

Community rehabilitation teams look after individuals once discharged from the unit and assist with reintegration into the community. Though, the frequency and intensity of therapy available in the community is far less than that available in inpatient rehabilitation units.

Inpatient Rehabilitation

Inpatient rehabilitation units can differ quite considerably in terms of their size, number of beds and access to therapies. Unfortunately, within the UK, access to rehabilitation is not uniform and services can vary significantly from area to area. However, all rehabilitation units have a number of common factors in their ethos:

- **They are multidisciplinary:** Therapists from different professional backgrounds work within the same rehabilitation unit. Whilst they will have variable strengths and areas of interest they work together as a team to provide the rehabilitation. The team will meet on a weekly basis to discuss progress.

- **Collaboration:** Rehabilitation is a collaborative exercise rather than a passive one. The patient will have to work together with their therapists to improve and maximise their function. Sometimes, a patient may be admitted to a rehabilitation unit and not yet be ready to partake fully in the process of rehabilitation. In those cases, the individual might need to go elsewhere until they are physically ready to go down the path of rehabilitation.

- **Goal planning:** Part of the process of individualised care and collaborative treatment, goals are agreed between the MDT and the individual. This is useful since it's best to rehabilitate the individual to perform tasks that they would have enjoyed doing in the past rather than new ones they'd have no interest in. For example, an elderly man might have no interest in getting rehabilitation to learn how to cook but might be more amenable to learning skills to do some gardening.

- **Individualised:** Rehabilitation is not a one size fits all form of therapy. No patient is the same, in terms of the size, scale, and location of the brain damage. No individual is similar in terms of their pre-injury background, personality or medical history. All of these factors strongly influence the process of rehabilitation.

- **Communication:** Good communication is a mainstay of rehabilitation and most rehabilitation units will attempt to facilitate this through regular meetings between the team and family members and the individual.

- **Less clinical:** Whilst many rehabilitation units are located on the grounds of hospitals, they are usually less clinical in their layout, decoration and structure. Bedrooms or bed areas are usually encouraged to be personalised with pictures or mementoes from home. Unlike traditional hospital wards, most patients will eat their meals along with other patients in a dining room area rather that at the bedside. Many, especially the newer units, are bright, airy and spacious with communal lounges to encourage inpatients to meet and socialise together.

- **Adapted:** Whilst on the surface inpatient rehabilitation wards look less clinical, they will have adaptations present to encourage mobilisation and reduce the risk of falls. Most will have grab rails located at the side of the wall for those who are unsteady on their feet. Bathrooms and toilets will usually have additional equipment for those in wheelchairs.

- **The importance of home:** During rehabilitation, many patients will have assessments in their home to see if any adjustments to stairs, bathrooms or bedroom location are required.

- **Planning:** Admissions and discharges are well planned in advance. Most rehabilitation units will have meetings prior to discharge. If the individual is being discharged to their own home they will spend regular weekends or nights at home before discharge to assess how they get on.

- **A process without an end:** Rehabilitation is a process that continues long after formal rehabilitation is complete. An individual with a brain injury will continue to improve on a gradual basis for many years. The speed of that recovery and rehabilitation is quicker and steeper early after the brain injury but ongoing improvements occur for some time after the completion of therapies.

The inpatient rehabilitation experience consists of three separate phases that overlap: an initial assessment phase, a therapies phase and a discharge planning phase.

Initial Assessment Phase

During the initial assessment phase, the therapists will assess the patient and determine their abilities and disabilities, their strengths and weaknesses. A physiotherapist might assess a patient's ability to walk or mobilise. An occupational therapist might assess the individual's abilities when washing, dressing, or preparing meals. A speech therapist will assess communication abilities and their ability to swallow. A psychologist or neuropsychiatrist might assess mood or cognition. Usually after these assessments are completed there will be a meeting between the therapy team, the individual and their family to feed back the results and to discuss the various goals of the inpatient stay and to ascertain the family's and individual's hopes and fears. This meeting also serves to answer any questions the individual or their family might have about the process.

Middle Therapy Phase

The middle therapy phase consists of achieving and reviewing goals based on the plans agreed at previous meetings. The individual goals are usually quite specific (e.g. to be able to stand up unassisted) and time limited. The middle phase is when most of the hard work between therapists and patient occurs. The duration of this phase varies considerably depending on the progress being made by the individual. The duration of this phase can also be influenced by local agreements about funding of rehabilitation.

Discharge Planning Phase

During this phase, the longer-term plans for the patient are discussed, planned and realised. This phase consists of meetings between the therapy team and family members and the individual to discuss the various options such as whether the individual will be able to return to their home or requires longer-term support.

Discharge Planning

The majority of individuals who suffer a brain injury return to their home after the acute phase of inpatient treatment and rehabilitation is complete. Most do not require additional support at home and informal additional help from family and friends will be enough.

Individuals who have mobility or other significant disabilities after a brain injury may require additional adaptations to their home for their own safety and to allow them to function more independently. This will usually be arranged prior to discharge by occupational therapists who will do a home visit with the patient and assess their ability to safely manage around their home. The adaptations required vary from simple ramps, stair rails, and rails in bathroom to reduce risk of falls, to more complicated adaptations of bathrooms and the kitchen.

The amount of support required when the individual is at home varies considerably from person to person depending on the severity of their injury, family circumstances, the layout of the house itself and the extent of any residual cognitive and behavioural problems. Support from external agencies varies greatly in terms of the number of visits per week and the duration of such visits. For those with milder problems, visits from a paid carer can last only a few minutes, a limited number of times per week. Those with more serious difficulties will require increased input, though due to cuts within the social care system arranging an appropriate level of care can be a challenge and the only other safe option left can mean the individual moving to a supervised flat, supported living or a care home.

Supervised or warden-controlled accommodation usually consists of the individual living in a complex that has a warden or person present at the entrance of the complex and is available for emergencies. The advantages of this are that there is support on hand in the event of problems but the individual retains a very high degree of independence. This option is fine for those with relatively little problems post-brain injury.

Supported living consists of the individual moving to a smaller group home where they will have a room of their own and share a kitchen and living room with other residents and carers that are present 24/7. This obviously has reduced independence but is still less institutionalised than a care home. The level of actual support within supported living facilities can vary considerably and just because there is someone on-site 24/7 doesn't mean that they will necessarily be available to be with the individual all or even part of the time. The agencies that operate such facilities usually operate on very thin margins and staff provision can be limited with poorly paid unskilled staff.

Survivors of brain injuries who require longer term care often can only receive it in care homes or nursing homes. The other residents in the majority of these will be far older and have dementias or physical health problems associated with older age. This can be socially quite difficult for the brain injury survivor. The levels of activities and level of cognitive stimulation available in such places is limited and the sum total of leisure activities may be restricted to watching television. This is hardly conducive to challenging, stimulating or improving overall cognitive abilities. However, long-term care options are expensive and care centres specifically set up for survivors of brain injuries are expensive to fund. Unfortunately, discharge options are significantly affected by the constrained social care funding available.

Increasingly, a considerable amount of care for individuals affected by severe brain injury with major behavioural and mental health problems is offered by private or so-called third sector specialist providers such as St Andrews, the Brain Injury Rehabilitation Trust or the Priory. These centres and centres like them offer longer-term care and support for individuals within their specialist units, which are located throughout the country. By their nature, they can be expensive but they offer a high degree of specialist support for individuals at the very severe end of the spectrum of behavioural problems.

FUNDING APPLICATIONS FOR LONGER-TERM CARE

The whole process of arranging funding to pay for the support packages is continually changing and is affected by the reduced levels of funds available to councils to pay for care in England and Wales. The system is quite complicated and can take a lot of time to navigate. The navigation is usually co-ordinated by a social worker.

In a nutshell, there are two major funding systems: social care and health funding. Most funding is provided through the local authority through social care funding. However, those with associated severe medical and behavioural problems and disabilities may be entitled to combine funding through the health services and the local authority. By its nature this funding source can fund more expensive packages, often in specialist centres, but the level of disability required to get such funding is high. The system of combined funding is slow and very bureaucratic and requires a lot of form filling by the treating team to present the request to a panel of often nameless professionals who decide on whether to fund the requested placement.

The bureaucracy associated with the processes can lead to delays in discharge from hospital and can be frustrating for the individuals, their families and treating teams. However, delays or no delays, the discharge destination and support present is an extremely important aspect of care for the individual and delays in adequate support shouldn't act as a reason to leave against medical advice.

TOP TIPS IN CARE HOME/SUPPORT FACILITY SECTION

In the preceding paragraphs, I have discussed how economic considerations means that in many, if not most cases, selection of care home facilities is based on monetary rather than purely clinical considerations. Care homes will all offer a certain degree of safety, and support the individual in their activities of daily living providing them with the basics of sustenance and some social interaction. However, individual nursing or care homes can differ significantly in terms of quality, training, expertise and ethos. Some care homes will be brand new and ultra-modern looking whereas other can look decidedly worn at the edges. Over my professional career I have visited many, and whilst the physical environment and the building itself is important, some care homes are decidedly more nurturing and welcoming than others and this is of utmost importance in the selection of any care home since first and foremost it is or should be a home for the individual. The wise family member should therefore try and look beyond the frayed carpets and see if the staff themselves are frayed!

In most cases, a family member will be informed of the care home or nursing home being selected. If they can at all, the family should try and visit the facility and meet with managers or staff. The following is a list of tips that are advisable when making the visit.

Prior to the visit, have a look at the care facility website and see what is promised in terms of facilities, activities, staffing and supports. Make a mental note of this and see how well aligned reality is to what is promised on the website.

Read any online reviews but be very mindful that individuals who write such reviews usually have a grievance against the facility and represent only a minority of experience and are usually extreme and frequently unhelpful.

For an objective opinion of the facility in England and Wales, read the reviews on the Care Quality Commission (CQC) website. These reviews are very detailed and offer an excellent and detailed assessment about the quality of the facility, staffing, management and the facilities safety.

Try not visit the facility alone but bring another friend or relative since two can always get a better opinion than just one on their own.

Arrange the appointment in advance so that you can meet with the manager or a nurse in charge. Unplanned visits are unfair and don't offer a necessarily better overview of the facility.

Have a well-prepared set of questions beforehand and in particular enquiry about:

- whether your loved one will have a room to themselves;
- the profile and ages of the other residents;
- the facility's experience of managing individuals with brain injuries.

If they state that they have input from physiotherapy, occupational therapy, psychology etc. ask them the amount of input they have and how often such therapists visit the facility. Some care/nursing homes boast on their website that they have therapists but actual availability of them is limited to a couple of hours per week or even less.

Do ask in detail about the activities that are offered – individuals with a brain injury need a certain degree of stimulation to improve clinically. All too often provision of activities is very limited. If it is the case that such activities are limited (and it frequently is) then as a family you'll need to supplement the lack of activities by visiting and taking the individual out if that is practical or safe.

Try and chat with the relatives of other residents who might be visiting at the same time. This can give a good idea about the nature of the quality of the facility.

Finally, be aware of your gut feeling and in particular whether it seems to be a caring place!

CASE HISTORY: THE MARATHON OF RECOVERY

Mark is a 25-year-old man who suffered a very severe brain injury after a motorbike accident. While riding his motorbike he was struck by a drunk driver. Mark was unconscious for a number of days and subsequently was confused for a number of weeks. In addition to a severe brain injury, he also sustained multiple broken bones. He required rehabilitation to help him walk again, and he needed a lot of input from speech therapy due to word-finding problems and slurred speech. He also required help from occupational therapists who helped him learn how to get washed and dressed again, and taught him how to become increasingly independent and to be able to care and cook for himself.

When he was discharged from a rehabilitation unit, he continued to require further community rehabilitation. His family felt that he worsened when he was discharged home, but the community rehabilitation team reminded his family that this was due to the fact that he was doing far more by himself at home than in the rehab unit. However, he continued to require considerable assistance on a day-to-day basis.

Due to the fact that his brain injury was the result of someone else's fault, he had a solicitor who started proceedings against the other driver and the other driver's insurance company. An interim case manager was appointed. Case managers come from a variety of healthcare backgrounds and are professionals that co-ordinate and purchase care privately. The case manager organised a package of care based around Mark's needs and funded by the interim payment made by the other driver's insurance company. The case manager organised for Mark to get extra assistance and support workers to come in during the week and help him go out. The case manager also managed to organise further additional rehabilitation with a physiotherapist, an occupational therapist and a speech therapist. Due to some anxiety that Mark developed around crossing roads, the case manager also organised some one-to-one psychology.

Even with all of this help, Mark continued to have his own challenges, although one of the benefits of the rehabilitation programme was that he was able to be more active in his community, and spend a couple of days a week doing a simple voluntary job. His sister, who had a company, also gave him a job for a couple of hours every week, sorting out letters and envelopes. This helped Mark get out of the house and it gave him a sense of achievement. Whilst he was able to live with a minimum of help, he continued to have his own challenges as a result of the brain injury.

This case history shows the complexity of rehabilitation and the ongoing nature of the recovery process. The package that someone like Mark has in this case study is impressive, and highlights the fact that individuals who have suffered a brain injury as a result of someone else's fault and where civil compensation proceedings are taking place frequently can have access to more intense comprehensive private rehabilitation packages. The fact that Mark's sister created a job in her office for him was particularly helpful. Whilst we all may be critical of our jobs on occasion, our jobs are far more than the source of our salary. Work gives people a sense of meaning. All of this is vital and of benefit in the chaotic circumstances that can occur after a brain injury.

The job is not so much a job in the employment sense as a form of rehabilitation and a psychological intervention in its own right.

CASE HISTORY: LIFE AFTER REHABILITATION

Kathleen suffered a severe brain haemorrhage in her 50s. As a result of this, she had reduced vision on one side and developed epilepsy. Whilst she lived with her husband and was able to do household chores and cook meals, she continued to have some memory challenges. She used simple techniques such as writing things down and keeping diaries to help her memory. She also had a large notice board in her kitchen, where she would pin bills that she had to pay, or other reminders. Her son, who is very technologically minded, also managed to programme an app on her phone to remind her to do various things. Many of her friends and neighbours who would meet her on the street thought that she was fully back to normal, and that it was like nothing had happened to her. However, Kathleen herself continued to feel that she was in some respects very different, although she was able to function reasonably well on a day-to-day basis.

This case history shows a common observation and frustration that many survivors of brain injuries complain of. They find that their family members can be indifferent to their ongoing cognitive and emotional challenges after the brain injury. Behind the scenes, a lot of additional support and assistance may be required. Use of aids such as notebooks, planners, noticeboards and newer phone reminders can be very helpful in such circumstances.

CHAPTER NINE

Unconsciousness, Coma, Low Awareness

DISORDERS OF CONSCIOUSNESS

Consciousness is defined as the state of having full awareness of what is going on and being able to react or respond to what is going on in one's environment. When we are asleep our level of consciousness is somewhat reduced but can readily return to normal when we wake up. Even whilst asleep we can quickly wake up if there is a lot of noise or if something dramatic happens in our surroundings.

We know what the absence of consciousness is but the nature of consciousness and the role of the brain involved in making us conscious remains a great mystery of science and philosophy. In daily life, most of us accept that we are conscious with little thought or understanding of what it means. It is usually only in encountering someone with reduced levels of consciousness or in a coma that one starts to realise how complex the whole concept actually is.

Death and Brain Death

Death is the ultimate state of unconsciousness. When someone is dead they don't respond to any stimuli, be it painful stimuli or loud noises. There is no electrical activity from the brain that can be measured using an EEG. There is no breathing and no beating of the heart. There are no spontaneous movements of the body. Reflexes are sudden and involuntary responses that our bodies make in response to a stimulus. When someone is brain dead such reflexes fail to happen. An

59

example of a reflex routinely tested to determine brain death is the corneal reflex when a wisp of cotton wool touches the cornea of the eye – normally this results in an immediate series of blinks. When the brain is dead, no such blinking occurs.

The development of ventilators and modern intensive-care technology has meant that for some patients it can be a challenge to determine whether they are alive or brain dead. This is an important distinction given that someone who is brain dead will not respond to any treatments and cannot recover. They are dead and only seem artificially alive due to the technology around them. A series of criteria have to be met to consider testing for brain death. These are that the individual does not have a reversible condition that will change or that they aren't unconscious due to hypothermia or medications. The individual's breathing can only be maintained by being on a ventilator. If these criteria are met, there should be no response to certain tests on neurological examination such as the constriction of the pupil in response to light. Brain death is established by different senior clinicians examining the individual on a number of occasions.

Individuals who are brain dead and on mechanical ventilation may be considered as suitable organ donors. On average a donor will donate 3.8 organs meaning that up to four individuals may have their lives transformed. However, many who are brain dead will not be considered suitable donors due to pre-existent medical conditions or due to physical complications as a result of their brain injury. A specialist organ donation nurse will liaise with medical team and family after the family have been informed that their loved one is brain dead. In such desperately difficult circumstances, the family will be approached by the nurse who discusses the options for organ donation and explain the process. In the devastating circumstances of death, organ donation and the knowledge that others have lived as a result of a loved one can give some degree of solace. Family refusal is a major obstacle towards organ donation. Most parts of the UK now have an opt-out system whereby all brain-dead patients are considered potential donors unless the individual previously recorded a decision not to donate.

Coma

A coma is the deepest level of unconsciousness in the living state, literally meaning 'deep sleep' in Greek. The heart still beats and lungs still breathe, though some individuals may require help with their breathing. Individuals in a coma don't have the cycle of waking and sleeping that is normally present. Instead they are unarousable and don't react to any stimuli such as noise or pain. The Glasgow Coma Scale (see chapter four) is a scale between 3 and 15 that assesses level of consciousness based on clinical examination. Ratings between 3 and 8 are considered to be indicative of a coma.

A prolonged coma is defined as a coma that lasts for more than 2 weeks. The longer the duration, the worse the outcome and the lower life expectancy is. Just half of those who remain in a coma a month after their brain injury will regain consciousness.

Frequently, individuals who are very confused and agitated and critically unwell are placed into a medically induced coma if they require assistance with breathing in intensive care. Medically induced comas are reversible when sedation is reduced or stopped.

In a coma the individual requires assistance with all of their nursing and medical needs. They are usually attached to a number of tubes including a urinary catheter which is a tube that is placed into the bladder to drain urine, a nasogastric tube to drain secretions from the stomach or provide the individual with a source of liquid food, or intravenous fluid drips to provide the individual with fluids or a means of giving the individual medications. Their breathing may be assisted through a tube that goes into the windpipe (or trachea) and pumps air into the lungs. The amount of tubes and assistance required varies greatly from individual to individual depending on the severity of their injuries.

Coma can be associated with a number of serious medical complications, many of which can be lethal. Infection is a serious risk that is always present and attempts are made to prevent severe infection by strict hygiene, monitoring temperature and treating any developing infection with antibiotics.

Bedsores are another risk and can easily develop due to the fact that the individual is lying down all the time. These can become infected and lead to septicaemia or blood poisoning as well as causing a lot of damage to the skin, sometimes requiring an operation to remove dead skin. The nursing staff monitor the health of skin closely and special air mattresses that circulate air to different parts of the body and reduce the amount of time an individual is lying in a particular position can prevent or minimise bedsores. Increasing levels of antibiotic resistance means that management of infection is becoming progressively more challenging. Clots are another potential complication and can develop in veins – usually leg veins. These clots can sometimes dislodge and migrate to the lungs where they cause a blockage in circulation and produce a pulmonary embolism that can be potentially fatal. The risk of clotting is reduced by giving an injection to thin the blood on a daily basis and also having the patient wear special stockings that compresses the veins in the leg.

The public perception of coma is often influenced by film portrayals. On television or the big screen, the end of a coma is often depicted as dramatically sudden with the individual waking up, fully alert and conscious and not confused. However, this isn't the case and most individuals will wake up, usually confused, only to go back into a coma some minutes later on a regular basis. The duration of being awake will increase gradually and the level of confusion usually diminishes with time.

Vegetative State

Vegetative state is the name given to a state where the individual appears to be awake or partially awake but has no awareness of what is going on around them. They are unable to purposely move their limbs or respond in any meaningful way to things around them except through simple reflexes. They will have a sleep–wake cycle with periods of being asleep and awake. However, during periods of being awake they will do little except lie with no real interaction towards people or things around them. They will display no evidence that they are aware of things going on around them or of their situation. They won't display any recognition of loved ones. In the immediate aftermath of waking from a coma, an individual can sometimes display reduced awareness. The longer the symptoms of reduced awareness last, the worse the outcome is. An individual who remains in a state of reduced awareness for more than a number of weeks is described as being in a persistent vegetative state. Persistent vegetative states are associated with catastrophic brain injuries and especially poor outcomes.

Minimally Conscious State

Minimally conscious state is the name given to when the individual is awake but has limited or minimal levels of awareness. The level of awareness can vary from being able to complete a few very simple movements to being able to use objects or follow commands or make sounds that can be understood.

In the initial stage, it can be difficult to distinguish between those who are in a vegetative state and in a minimal conscious state. However, it is important to distinguish between them since those with minimal consciousness have a somewhat better outcome. Therapists may use a series of simple tests repeated a number of times per day over a number of weeks to determine whether the individual can respond to stimuli in their environment. One example of such a test that is popularly used in the UK is SMART. The SMART or Sensory Modality Assessment and Rehabilitation Technique is a highly structured set of tests that was developed at the Royal Hospital for Neurodisability in London. It can also be used to assess if an individual can communicate with others by methods such as blinking or moving various parts of the head or body. The examination is standardised and the therapist doing the assessment uses a variety of clinical tests to see if the individual can respond or react to different stimuli including sound, images, touch, smell or taste. A patient who is able to react on a regular basis is, by definition, not in a vegetative state.

Locked-in Syndrome

Large bleeds or damage to parts of the brain stem can leave the individual unable to move or speak but fully able to hear and understand what is going on around them. This distressing state is described as being locked in and was poignantly described in the book *The Diving Bell and Butterfly* by French journalist Jean-Dominique Bauby who developed the syndrome after a stroke. Individuals with locked-in syndrome can communicate, albeit with difficulty, through blinking their eyes or using other eye movements. Speech therapists have a particularly important role in assisting individuals with this condition, and new computer eye-tracking devices can allow the individual to communicate one letter at a time.

DISORDERS OF CONSCIOUSNESS AND THE FAMILY

Disorders of consciousness are particularly stressful for families and the ordeal of waiting can feel like an emotional rollercoaster. The waiting for a coma to end can be particularly trying and the tendency of patients to have fluctuating levels of consciousness can be frustrating when they appear to be more alert one day only to be less conscious the next. During this time, there can also be lots of medical problems and difficulties. The environment within an intensive care unit is far from ideal and can come across as very clinical and impersonal. This, combined with frequently restrictive visiting hours and the sheer level of uncertainty associated with outcome at this stage, can make it very stressful for family members. The period of time when the individual is in a coma is essentially a waiting game and it can be very easy to cling to vestiges of hope only to be deflated the next day.

General Advice for Families

• If you come from a large family, try to establish a rota for visits rather than turning up en masse to intensive care units. Visitor restrictions are in place as much for the safety of the loved one as for other patients since visitors bring germs.

- Do not visit if you have an infection or are suffering from any bug or gastroenteritis. In particular if you have had diarrhoea or vomiting in the previous 72 hours, keep away!

- Be aware of hand hygiene regulations on the unit and follow them very carefully – individuals in ITU are very vulnerable to getting infections. Rates of antibiotic-resistant bacteria are rising in the community and represent a serious challenge for hospitals. Prevention of infection through scrupulous hand hygiene is essential.

- Try not to blame medical and nursing staff for slowness of your loved one coming out of a coma. In the highly distressed and frustrated state of waiting for a sign of the coma to end, it can be very easy to project one's fear and annoyance into anger towards others. Ultimately, the medical and nursing staff are trying to achieve the same outcome as you are.

- Try to be open to bad news – medical staff will attempt to inform family members of bad news in as sensitive a manner as possible. However, even with the best of intentions it is possible for miscommunication to occur and for family members to get upset and annoyed if information relating to outcome is less positive than hoped.

- In cases of vegetative state, it can be easy to misinterpret normal reflexes or spontaneous non-purposeful movements as signs of an attempt to communicate with the world. If you do believe that your loved one is responding to you, let therapists know.

- Be aware of your own mental and physical health and seek help if required. Visiting a loved one in a coma or state of reduced awareness can be enormously draining, both emotionally and physically, particularly when there is little change on a day-to-day basis.

- Be sensitive to the possibility that even if a loved one appears to have reduced consciousness that they may have some understanding, especially if there's a chance that they might have locked-in syndrome. Therefore, try not to say overly negative or derogatory things in front of them.

- Do talk to your loved one – whether you believe they can hear you or not.
- Be open to taking a day off from visiting in order to do housework, pay bills, attend to other family members and recharge. The whole process through recuperation after a brain injury is a marathon and not a sprint. Burned out and exhausted family members are no good to anyone – least of all their loved one.

CASE HISTORY: LOCKED-IN SYNDROME

Jonathan was a healthy 58-year-old father of three grown-up children. He had been diagnosed some years previously with high blood pressure, but he didn't take his blood pressure medication. He kept busy and was always working hard in his role as a builder. However, one day he collapsed at work, and was unresponsive. He was transferred to the local hospital, and a brain scan showed a large bleed at the back of the brain. He was treated for some time in intensive care.

He was eventually transferred to the main ward, but remained unresponsive. Although he appeared to be awake and had his eyes open, he was unable to move any of his four limbs, or talk, or move his head. Very early on, his medical team told the family about the severity of his bleed and resulting brain injury. The team initially wondered whether he might be in a persistent vegetative state. As a result, he was seen by a speech and language therapist. She tested him using a variety of methods before she realised that he was able to respond through blinking his left eye. Though communication from Jonathan was extremely difficult and slow. The speech and language therapist would go through the alphabet and get him to blink his eye when they reached a letter or word he wanted to communicate. Using this technique, she very slowly and laboriously was able to demonstrate that he knew what was going on around him. With some time, she managed to train his family in learning how to communicate with him, using the same technique. However, any form of communication was very strenuous.

This case history tells a story that is desperately distressing for the individual and their family. Cases like this are a living nightmare and ordeal for everyone concerned. Technology in terms of assisting with communication remains at best, in early stages of development at present. It is to be hoped that new technologies will facilitate easier communication in the future.

CASE HISTORY: PERSISTENT VEGETATIVE STATE

Patrick was a 21-year-old mechanic. He liked nothing better than cars, and had a tendency to drive too fast. He was involved in a serious accident while speeding. In addition to multiple fractures throughout his body, he suffered catastrophic brain injuries. He had bleeding throughout his brain, as well as bruising on the frontal lobes, and his treating team believed that he also had diffuse axonal injury.

Due to his fractures, he required a number of operations and was treated for many weeks in intensive care, where he was sedated. The sedation was slowly withdrawn and he began to open his eyes. However, clinicians noted that he was quite unresponsive to commands, even though his eyes were open and he seemed awake. When he was transferred to a rehabilitation unit, he received some input from speech therapy and occupational therapy. He needed full nursing care, and was unable to eat, drink or swallow, and so he received food via a special feeding tube. Whilst he appeared to be awake at times, and asleep at other times, he did not appear to respond to anyone around him, or recognise anyone around him, and the treating team wondered if he was in a persistent vegetative state.

As a result, a speech therapist completed a SMART assessment. After completion of the extensive assessment, her opinion was that he was in a persistent vegetative state.

CHAPTER TEN

Post-traumatic Amnesia (PTA)

Contrary to what is portrayed in films or some television soaps, when someone wakes up after being in a coma they are very rarely able to recall the circumstances of their injury – much less how it happened or who caused it. Any brain injury causing a coma for more than 24 hours is by definition severe. Memory of events leading up to the brain injury will be lost or at the very least muddled. This form of memory loss is called retrograde amnesia. The amount of memories lost leading up to the time of the brain injury can vary from person to person; people can occasionally report no recollection of anything for weeks prior to a brain injury, though most will report no recollection for minutes to hours.

On waking up after being in a coma, most are confused and disorientated. This disorientation can continue for quite a while depending on the severity of the brain injury. In the case of very mild brain injuries, this confusion may be absent or last less than 24 hours. However, in more severe injuries, the confusion may last days, weeks, months or indefinitely. This confusion and disorientation is called post-traumatic amnesia (PTA). During this period, the individual will be unable to register new information despite being told what is happening to them. The actual cause is unclear but brain wave tests show that the brain is working slower than normal.

Confusion can take the form of being disorientated in time, meaning the individual is unaware of the day, date, month, season, or year. They may be disorientated in place, meaning that they may be unaware of where they are. They will have no understanding as to why they are in hospital or what has happened to them.

In the case of PTA, this confusion persists despite being repeatedly told by family and staff where they are or the presence of a whiteboard beside the bed displaying the day and location. They will be unaware of their injury or of any input from rehabilitation therapists or hospital staff or of any family visits or things said during those visits. Family members will notice their loved one will ask the same set of questions over and over again and have limited understanding of what is going on around them.

Often confusion is associated with agitation, meaning that the individual may try to get out of bed or leave the hospital despite being advised that this is unwise. They will lack insight and may trivialise the extent of their injury and dismiss that they have any difficulties. They may report a strong desire to leave the healthcare facility and return to their home or return to work despite the fact that this would be clearly unwise. The resulting agitation when they are stopped from leaving the ward can take the form of shouting at staff, threats of physical violence or actual violence against staff. Some may settle with gentle reassurance or through distracting techniques, e.g. saying that a family member will be in later to visit them or asking them to talk about their family or hobbies prior to their injury. Many in acute care facilities will require the presence of a staff member to stay with them at all times to reassure and remind them where they are and the reason for being there.

Occasionally, the level of agitation may be so severe that the individual may be violent and hurt themselves or others due to the level of their distress and no amount of reassurance from staff will suffice. In these cases, the individual may require medication in the form of tranquilisers to make them more relaxed and reduce the risk of absconding or causing harm to themselves or others. The types of tranquillisers used vary from hospital to hospital. However, they are usually given at as low a dose as will be effective for the patient. The types of medication used include benzodiazepines such as lorazepam or diazepam – these are very safe if given in small doses for a short period of time. Anti-psychotic medications also have an ability to make the patient more relaxed and less distressed and again are often used in cases of agitation. Whilst staff in hospitals like to give as little medications as possible after a brain injury, allowing a person after a brain injury to be distressed, upset, agitated and potentially violent is unkind as well as potentially dangerous for the individuals.

Sometimes during this period of confusion, the individual may be so confused that they say very hurtful and upsetting things to family members. It is advisable to try and not take any upsetting things said personally since the individual is not their usual selves during this time and isn't in control of their emotions or how they react.

The experience of being in PTA and being confused can be extremely scary and distressing for the sufferer. We can liken it to the feeling we have when we are having a scary dream; when young children become confused with a temperature; or when someone is extremely drunk. I have encountered families who were so upset with what their relative said during their confusion that they sought to subsequently discuss what was said with them. This is a pointless exercise that is upsetting for both parties and is akin to reminding someone what they said in their sleep.

Coming out of PTA/confusion is a gradual process. The time it takes to fully emerge from that confusion varies a lot depending on the severity of the injury, age of the individual and any other physical health issues. The first sign is that the individual is mildly less confused – that is to say, they may be unaware of the day, month or year but are able to say what city they are in or the name of the institution. That level of awareness can fluctuate with time or level of fatigue. It is usual for someone to be more confused later in the day or evening time when reduced lighting can lead to further disorientation. However, over a period of days or weeks that level of fluctuating confusion gets less and less, so that they can gradually say what day, date, month it is and where they are and what happened to them. Health issues like a urinary tract infection or even constipation can lead to temporary steps backwards and the individual becoming more confused again. Time is the key to resolving the physical problems within the brain leading to the confusion and it is unlikely that any intervention from either family or hospital team can shorten that duration.

The period spent waiting for or hoping for emergence from confusion can be a lonely and scary one for the family. It can frequently be a case of one step forward and two steps back. Combined with this is the sense of fear that the individual might not ever emerge from their confusion – particularly when weeks gradually pass with limited improvements. Medical professionals can never definitively answer when or if the confusion may end and there can be a general sense of frustration with the pace of progress. Information is limited during this period and not infrequently can be contradictory. There can also be a sense of being at an impasse since acute treatment of surgical and medical problems may have stopped and the loved one remains confused.

General Advice for Families

In terms of general advice on visiting etc. please see chapter nine.

- Regular visiting can be really helpful in orientating the individual and lessening their distress.
- Some hospitals encourage family to help with aspects of the individual's nursing care, such as helping them with repositioning pillows, hand care, assisting with their walking, oral care and shaving. The list varies from hospital to hospital and can be influenced by infection control measures.
- During visits if the individual is particularly agitated try and distract them through music, reading or watching the television or DVDs with them.
- If family members are finding it difficult to know what to discuss, reminiscence about happy past holidays, adventures or events is very helpful.
- Bringing in photos or valued (not valuable!) personal mementos can also help but please discuss with nursing staff first.
- Advise care staff about the individual's background, their likes and dislikes, hobbies and topics of interest. It can be very useful for family to write these out and give a copy to nursing staff.

CASE HISTORY: POST-TRAUMATIC AMNESIA

Harriet was a 54-year-old woman with a secret drinking problem. One night when she had drunk too much alcohol, she slipped and fell down the stairs. A neighbour found her the next morning in an unconscious state. She was transferred to hospital and found to have a skull fracture, some bleeding on the brain, and bruising to the brain. She was unconscious for a number of days and was very confused on regaining consciousness. Family members would come in to visit her and she would tell them that she was at home in her living room. She believed her sons were her brothers, and similarly would confuse one of her daughter's as being her mother. She had no idea what day, month or even year it was.

Her family used visit her with a sense of apprehension as to what her behaviour would be like on the day. Some days she would be pleasantly confused, and on other days she would be irritable, nasty and tell them quite hurtful things. The staff who were looking after her on the ward would report that she was up at night-time and asleep during the daytime.

This is a classic history of someone in post-traumatic amnesia. Their level of consciousness varies on an hour-by-hour and day-to-day basis. With time, such confusion may become less and the situation will normalise. However, in the case of individuals like Harriet, when alcohol abuse has been an issue, the clinical presentation can be complicated by alcohol-related brain damage. That damage can take the form of severe short-term memory problems due to damage of the parts of the brain that encode new information. People like Harriet can therefore develop chronic problems with learning and recalling of new information.

CHAPTER ELEVEN

Physical Problems After a Brain Injury

SPEECH AND COMMUNICATION PROBLEMS

Dysphasia is term for speech problems as a result of damage to the brain. The process of speaking is a complex one which involves the larynx, pharynx, lungs and multiple parts of the brain. Damage to these structures or anywhere along the pathways between them can result in varying forms of speech problems. Similarly, other factors such as fatigue, pain, medications, hearing or general confusion may affect the quality of communication.

At its most basic, the process of communication can be considered to be comprised of two major elements: a sensory element that understands what others are saying and a motor element that converts the thoughts that the individual wants to express into the co-ordinated physical movements to produce articulated speech. Both of these elements are controlled by the so-called 'dominant' part of the brain. This is the left hemisphere of the brain in right-handed people and right hemisphere in many people who are left-handed.

The motor element involved in speech production is called Broca's area. The sensory element is called Wernicke's area. Different forms of brain injuries can dramatically affect speech if either part of the brain is damaged. Damage to parts of the cerebellum and brain stem can also affect the ability to speak. The most common cause of damage to either area is through strokes, bleeds or aneurysms.

Damage to Broca's area is more often observed – especially after a stroke – and produces a problem with speech called an expressive

73

dysphasia, also called motor dysphasia or telegraphic speech. An individual with an expressive dysphasia will understand fully what others are saying and know what they want to say but the correct words will not come out. As a result, the speech can be broken or disjointed. The individual affected will be fully aware that the words coming out are not what they want to say and as a result can be very frustrated, upset and tearful. The risk of development of depression is particularly high in people affected with this type of speech problem. Fortunately, a mixture of time and speech therapy can help greatly; however, many may be left with residual ongoing speech and word-finding problems. Use of picture charts can help some to communicate better. Family members can quickly become used to some of the speech patterns and understand what the individual means to say despite the fact that the speech is disjointed. Encouraging the individual to speak slower and more clearly can also help since word finding problems are far worse if the individual speaks too fast.

Damage to Wernicke's area produces a sensory dysphasia or receptive dysphasia. Fortunately, this happens less often than a motor dysphasia. In a sensory dysphasia the individual misinterprets what others are saying to them. Their speech will appear fluent but will be nonsensical. They will be unaware of the fact that others don't understand them. On hospital wards in the acute setting they can appear very confused or agitated but this is usually due to the fact that they have no understanding of what is going on around them. As a family member, it can be difficult to cope with this form of dysphasia and it is advisable to offer the individual gentle reassurance and try and use simple language with lots of non-verbal body language to communicate.

If an individual has damage to the back part of the brain, they can develop a speech problem similar to that seen in someone who is drunk. The individual will be able to talk but the words come out poorly articulated and sound slurred, nasal and monotonous. It can be difficult at first to follow what is being said, especially if there is associated word-finding difficulties. This form of speech problem can be seen in a wide variety of other neurological disorders including Huntington's disease, multiple sclerosis and motor neuron disease. One of the problems associated with it is that the general public can judge individuals with this speech pattern and think that they are intoxicated. I have encountered horror stories of people with brain injuries being refused to board a bus due their slurring speech. This can lead to the individual being very self-conscious and avoiding going out socially.

General Advice for Speech Problems

- Encourage the individual affected to talk slowly.
- As a family member, don't be afraid to ask your loved one to repeat themselves – the more they repeat themselves the better their speech gets and the better your ability to understand them becomes.
- Don't interrupt or finish sentences for them – firstly, it annoys the individual and secondly, is stops them from learning and practicing.
- Try and be patient and use non-verbal communication with body language.
- Listen carefully to what is being said – with practice it is possible to become proficient in understanding the new speech patterns of the individual and what they are trying to communicate.
- For those with slurred speech it is possible to obtain an ID type card from Headway, the brain injury charity, that says they have had a brain injury. This can be used when in shops or social situations to left staff and public know that the individual has a brain injury and is not intoxicated.
- If in doubt get advice from speech therapy – they are usually more than happy to offer advice and guidance.

SWALLOWING PROBLEMS

Swallowing difficulties, called dysphagia, can commonly occur after a brain injury for a number of reasons. The whole process of swallowing requires the co-ordinated efforts of a number of parts of the brain and muscles within the mouth, throat, and gullet (oesophagus). Damage to the frontal lobes or parts of the brainstem can damage that ability to co-ordinate things or can affect the individual's ability to concentrate appropriately to complete the complex task. Lying down all the time or being in the wrong position can also make it harder and sometimes after being unconscious for a while, the muscles themselves can lose their tone and be less efficient in their task.

Swallowing problems are serious and not just an inconvenience. At its most severe, food can go into the lungs instead of the stomach and cause the individual to choke or become very unwell with an aspiration pneumonia. At a minimum, swallowing problems are associated with coughing, spluttering, wheezing and spitting-out food/drink when trying to swallow. It's unpleasant and upsetting for the patient, however those with very severe brain injuries who lack insight may not understand the connection between swallowing food and choking and can potentially endanger their lives if they get access to food.

A swallowing assessment by a speech therapist is a potentially life-saving test given the hazards of food going down the wrong way. The assessment needs to be performed before an individual is declared safe to eat or drink. In most hospitals, a sign above the bed will say whether food or fluids can be consumed orally by the patient. If oral intake is not allowed, then it is really important not to give the individual anything by mouth even if they are demanding food or drink. Wet swabs can be used to moisten the lips but breaking the rules and giving food potentially endangers the health of the individual and can lead to safeguarding concerns being made.

An individual with severe swallowing problems who is unable to eat or drink can obtain their nutritional requirements in other ways. Nasogastric feeding involves inserting a small feeding tube into the nose and down the oesophagus (or gullet) and into the stomach. The position of the tube is checked by X-ray and a bag of a liquid feed is attached and slowly administered overnight or over a period of hours. Nasogastric feeding is a short-term solution. For those with longer-term feeding problems a tube is inserted into the stomach under general anaesthetic. This form of feeding is called percutaneous endoscopic gastrostomy (PEG) or enteral feeding.

When there is some ability to swallow, the safety of swallowing can be improved by thickening the consistency of foods and fluids. However, some individuals may require the addition of food thickeners to water and other liquid foods. These thickeners turn the food into a jelly-like or wallpaper paste-like semi-solid texture. Theoretically they are tasteless, however, most people don't enjoy having to use thickeners especially for liquids like tea or coffee.

General Advice for Swallowing Problems

- Carefully follow the advice given by speech therapy or nursing staff – if oral intake is banned then do not bring in sweets or foods behind the backs of staff.
- Try to encourage someone with a brain injury to eat sitting up in an area that is free from distraction and noise.
- Encourage smaller meals and don't overload the plate with food. For those with frontal lobe problems who are at risk of stuffing their mouths, monitor intake and avoid leaving them beside large boxes of biscuits, sweets etc.
- If you notice any coughing, spluttering or evidence that food is going down the wrong way, tell staff and remove the food from the individual.

BALANCE

Balance is the ability to be upright without toppling and falling over. Dizziness is the name given to the sensation that the individual or the world is swaying or spinning – it can in itself cause balance difficulties or result from balance problems. Balance is quite an underrated and surprisingly complicated mechanism involving coordination between a number of different parts of the body and different parts of the brain. Problems with steadiness lead to difficulty with sitting up, standing up and walking and results in falls. Individuals with the most severe forms of balance problems are incapable of safely mobilising on their own and will frequently require wheelchairs.

Due to the fact that a number of different parts of the brain are involved in stability, damage to any one of these areas can result in balance problems.

When an individual is bed bound for a prolonged period of time they become weak due to muscle bulk loss. The body's blood pressure mechanism also is affected as the body starts to get used to being flat. The mechanisms that automatically take place every morning when we get up from a lying down position fail and as a result the blood pressure drops and the individual feels weak and they get a sensation of dizziness when they try to raise their head above the pillow. Physiotherapists and nurses can treat this by gently raising the angle of the head on a progressive basis over a period of days to weeks and bit by bit getting them to sit up and eventually stand up. Exercises and stretches are used to progressively improve muscle strength and stamina so that the individual can stand.

Individuals who aren't bed bound can suffer from a sensation of dizziness and develop balance problems due to damage or irritation to balance sense organs that exist within the ear. This balance sense, or vestibular system organ, consists of three tiny semi-circular canals that are orientated at 90 degrees to each other. In normal circumstances the stimulation of one set of canals at a particular angle relative to the other allows the brain to work out the position of the head . After a head injury, this very delicate organ can be damaged by small pieces of debris in the canals which gives the individual the sensation that their head is in a different position to where the eyes and other ear is saying it is. This disconnect in information creates a sensation of dizziness and causes balance issues. Physiotherapists are able to move that small piece of grit out of the canals and reduce the imbalance through getting the individual to reposition their head in certain ways.

The brain centrally processes the information it receives from those semi-circular canals and other position sensors that are located in muscles throughout the body. The cerebellum, located at the back of the brain, processes this information and uses it to adapt fine movement so that it is more co-ordinated. The cerebellum can be damaged directly due to trauma or as a result of medication or drugs. The unsteadiness seen in individuals who are drunk is, in part, due to the effect of alcohol on this part of the brain.

Balance problems may also result from neglect of one side of the body. Damage to the frontal lobes means that the individual's ability to plan movement is impaired so that they move impulsively and unwisely. Attention problems may mean that they aren't able to respond to sudden changes in movement required.

TINNITUS

Tinnitus is a distressing sense of hearing a buzzing, ringing, hissing or other sound in the ears in the absence of an external cause. One or both ears may be affected. Traumatic brain injury is just one of many causes – others include ear damage, wax build-up, sinusitis or tumours. Like dizziness, it is seen in all levels of traumatic brain injury and is frequently seen in post-concussion syndrome. It may have many causes but is usually due to some degree of damage or irritation of the sensitive hearing structures of the ears from a trauma. Many individuals find it very distressing and it can affect sleep and be a cause of anxiety and depression.

Treatment of tinnitus is generally dependent on the cause but it responds poorly to medications, though sedatives and antidepressants are regularly used and can help greatly with associated anxiety or sleep problems. Cognitive behavioural therapy (CBT) and relaxation therapy are also used in its management with various degrees of success. Regular meditation and having background noise are also excellent ways of improving quality of life associated with the symptoms. In most cases, it improves with time. Individuals with tinnitus in particular should be wary of reading online forums related to the condition. These forums often present worse case scenarios and can be more of a source of stress than the tinnitus itself.

MOBILITY PROBLEMS

The ability to walk after a brain injury can be affected due to a long list of causes. Direct damage to the brain, the balance centres or damage to the limbs themselves can all severely affect mobility.

Fractures, dislocations or sprains to limbs as a result of the trauma that led to the brain injury can obviously affect whether an individual can walk and the quality of their mobilisation. Prolonged immobility due to being bed bound causes weakening of muscles remarkably quickly. Dizziness and balance problems can also adversely affect the individual's confidence to get out and walk.

Mobilisation within the brain is initiated, controlled and modified by a number of structures. Movements are initiated by the motor cortex in the frontal lobes, with the left motor cortex controlling movement on the right side of the body and vice versa. Damage to the motor cortex will produce paralysis or weakness on the opposite side. This part of the brain can be damaged in strokes, bleeds or as a result of localised trauma.

The cerebellum at the back of the brain has an important role in facilitating fine movement and it can be directly damaged due to trauma or bleeds or temporarily affected due to drugs or toxins. Damage to the spinal cord can also affect mobilisation by causing paralysis.

As we discussed earlier, physiotherapists are required to improve mobility Occupational therapists will work with physiotherapists in coming up with solutions to improve mobility through use of walking aids, walking sticks or wheelchairs. However, given the multitude of causes of difficulties and influence of other factors such as prolonged immobility, improvements take time and requires patience and a collaborative approach by both the patient and therapists.

EPILEPSY

Neurons within the brain communicate through a form of electrical discharges from neuron to neuron. Those discharges are coordinated and well controlled. A seizure is the name given to episodic uncontrolled electrical activity of the brain. The uncontrolled electrical activity can result in various symptoms such as limb shaking, altered awareness or behavioural changes.

Epilepsy is diagnosed when a person is prone to having recurrent seizures. Seizures can broadly be divided into two types: focal and generalised. Focal seizures result from damage to a particular part of the brain – most commonly the temporal lobe. Generalised seizures represent episodes of abnormal electrical activity throughout the brain. Focal, or partial seizures, can be described as 'simple', where someone's awareness isn't affected. Simple focal seizures may take the form of a limb or other part of the body having uncontrolled movements.

Complex Partial Seizure

More commonly, the awareness of the individual is affected and during the seizure they become unaware of what's going on around them. This is called complex a partial seizure and are often associated with an aura, which is a set of sensations that occur just before the onset. The symptoms associated with the aura depends on the part of the brain affected; in the case of temporal lobe epilepsy, these symptoms can include a smelling burning, a metallic taste, alterations in one's vision, abdominal sensations or a sensation of panic or anxiety. The individual then loses consciousness and may start shaking or have other symptoms.

Generalised Epilepsy

Generalised epilepsy may be associated with absences – formerly called petit mals – where the individual stares into space or goes blank for a period of time without any collapse. They can be very subtle and frequently can be misinterpreted by others who think that the individual is just daydreaming.

Tonic-clonic

Tonic-clonic or grand mal seizures are far more dramatic and scary for family members. These fits have three separate phases. The first phase is called a tonic phase due to the fact that the individual goes stiff and rigid. The seizure starts off with loss of consciousness. The person stops breathing, goes stiff and rigid and falls to the ground. During this phase, their lips or face may go blue due to lack of oxygen. This phase then ends with the individual gasping and starting to shake. The clonic phase starts and limbs will be observed shaking for a number of minutes. This phase may be associated with the individual involuntarily wetting themselves or biting their tongue. After the shaking ends the individual enters the post-ictal phase where they may remain asleep for a few minutes and on gaining consciousness they will be tired and confused and complain of sore muscles and limbs.

In the immediate aftermath of a brain injury or head trauma, an individual may have a seizure. Not everyone will have further seizures and develop epilepsy, however many will. The risk of epilepsy is particularly high in those with head injuries in which the skull is penetrated by a foreign body, for example a knife or other piece of metal. The chance is somewhat lower in those whose skull wasn't breached. The potential of developing epilepsy can remain increased for many years after a moderate to severe brain injury.

Diagnosis and Treatment

Epilepsy is usually diagnosed by a neurologist. They may use electro-encephalography (EEG) or a brain wave test to assist with diagnosis, particularly if the seizure sounds unusual. EEGs are usually performed briefly over a period of an hour or so. However, in some cases, the individual may have the electrodes attached to the scalp and a mobile device and be sent home for 24 to 48 hours in the hope that they have a seizure during that time. Occasionally an individual may be admitted to hospital for a period of a few days to have an EEG whilst in a room with cameras to record the actual seizure. Doctors may sometimes try to bring on a seizure when someone is attached to an EEG by reducing the anti-epileptic medication or by depriving them of sleep. This is because capturing a seizure whilst an individual is linked up to an EEG machine is very useful clinically. The EEG will pick up any changes in the brain waves and can be used to determine where the seizure is coming from and the types of treatment indicated.

There are a number of different anti-epileptic drugs (AEDs) available. Some are more effective than others and different AEDs can vary considerably in their side effects. Some of them – such as phenytoin – can interact with other medications and their levels in the blood can become too high and can be associated with severe side effects. As a result, phenytoin may require blood tests to check levels within the blood. Other AEDs like carbamazepine can be associated with lowering the levels of sodium in the blood causing dizziness and confusion. Valproate can affect liver function blood tests. In the context of brain injury, however, both valproate and carbamazepine are also used for reducing agitation and stabilising mood. It's always worth carefully reading the list of side effects associated with different AEDs and being aware of potential other medications to avoid taking with them.

Unfortunately, despite amount of AEDs available, up to 40 % of sufferers will have a form of epilepsy that doesn't respond well to medications. Various combinations of tablets can be used to try and reduce the frequency of seizures.

Epilepsy is also associated with increased rates of mental health problems like depression, anxiety and, occasionally, psychosis. These mental health problems may be due to the unpredictable nature of epilepsy itself or occasionally due to the anti-epileptic drugs.

Not uncommonly, some of the seizures that a patient presents with may be stress related and not due to electrical problems within the brain. These stress-related seizures have a variety of names including non-epileptic seizures, non-epileptic attack disorder, dissociative seizures, psychogenic non-epileptic seizures, or pseudoseizures. Investigation using an EEG or videos of the apparent seizures can be particularly useful in their diagnosis. Accurate diagnosis can be a challenge in such cases but is important since patients with stress-related seizures require psychiatric treatment and not more anti-epileptic medications.

To complicate matters further, individuals with epilepsy can also present with non-epileptic seizures.

General Advice for Epilepsy

- During a seizure do not attempt to put a spoon or any object into the mouth of the individual having the seizure. The myth about swallowing one's tongue during a seizure is an old wives' tale and should be disregarded as teeth have been seriously damaged due to this practice.

- The best thing to do during a seizure is to clear the area of furniture or other objects around the individual having the seizure so that they don't hurt themselves. When the seizure is complete try and place the individual into the recovery position.

- Try to be aware of how long the seizure is going on and seek medical help or call an ambulance if it is not stopping, if the seizure is a first seizure or is different to usual seizures.

- After the seizure is finished encourage the individual to rest if they are tired and if they're confused gently remind them where they are.

- For individuals with diagnosed epilepsy, try to monitor the seizure frequency by noting them in a diary. Some neurologists will routinely give out a seizure diary to their patients and it is useful to bring this to clinic.

- In the cases of unusual-looking or new seizure presentations, it can be very useful if the family video the seizure using a mobile phone and show this to neurologists or doctors at clinics. This may not feel like a nice thing to do at the time, but it is very helpful for doctors and aids diagnosis.

- Seizures can be triggered in some individuals through alcohol, fatigue or strobe lighting. It's useful to minimise these if they are known risk factors for provoking a seizure.

- Mental health problems are particularly common with epilepsy so it is useful to be aware of the potential to develop such difficulties and inform your doctor if this is the case. It is not uncommon for psychiatric complications associated with epilepsy to be more disabling than the epilepsy itself.

- Driving with uncontrolled epilepsy is not permitted and as well as being potentially lethal to other road users is a prosecutable offence. Individuals who have driven despite having epilepsy have been sent to prison. The duration of time an individual is required to be seizure free differs considerably from jurisdiction to jurisdiction. If one has been seizure-free and wishes to start driving again please discuss with your neurologist before going behind the wheel, and in the UK inform the DVLA.

Valproate or valproic acid should be avoided in women who might become pregnant as its use can be associated with damage to the foetus and birth defects. Women on this medication should use contraception if they are sexually active and speak with their physicians if they are thinking of becoming pregnant. Women on other anti-epileptic medications who are of childbearing years or planning on getting pregnant should also discuss their medications with their treating doctor.

SPASTICITY AND CONTRACTURES

There are two basic types of paralysis: one associated with the limb being floppy and the other associated with the limb being rigid.

The second, rigid type of paralysis is due to damage of the nerves anywhere along its path from the brain down through the neck and into the spine. It may be seen after a stroke or bleed. It is also called upper motor neuron damage. The limbs affected with this form of paralysis aren't floppy and instead are tight and may be passively moved by others only with difficulty. In upper motor neuron damage, the arms have a tendency to adopt a flexed position and can be bent at the elbow and are difficult to straighten. In contrast, the legs have a tendency to be extended and completely straightened. With time and in the absence of regular physiotherapy and exercises the affected limbs can become fixed and difficult to move or spastic.

Such spasticity can mean that simple everyday tasks such as washing, putting on clothes and even sitting can become difficult to perform for carers. With time the individual can develop contractures to the point that the individual affected limb cannot be passively moved by others at all.

The exact cause of spasticity is unknown and some individuals appear to be more prone to it than others. In the rehabilitation setting it can be prevented through input from a number of therapists. Physiotherapists and nursing staff can help reduce its development through use of passive exercises where the therapist will gently move the affected limb repeatedly to reduce the level of tightness. Such exercise may need to be performed daily, however even with this, some will continue to become stiffer and require additional interventions. Occupational therapists can reduce spasticity and contractures through making splints to keep an affected limb in a particular position. Splints are usually made of plastic and can be obtained either off the shelf or made/modified for the individual's needs. Splints are usually used overnight or for prolonged periods of time when a limb may be immobile and not being stretched. They can be uncomfortable to wear and unpopular with the individual though they have an important role in the prevention of development of contractures.

The rehabilitation doctor also has a role in the management of spasticity through use of medications or other interventions. Baclofen is one medication which promotes muscle relaxation that is regularly used in spasticity. This drug is most usually given orally but it is associated with a number of side effects, the most important being drowsiness and occasionally agitation or anxiety. Infrequently, it can be given directly into the spine – called intrathecally – and administered regularly using a pump. This form of administration is less commonly used and only attempted when oral baclofen doesn't work.

Other medications that are commonly used include gabapentin or pregabalin or medications from the benzodiazepines group such as diazepam or clonazepam.

In more localised spasticity a poison called botulinum toxin (commonly called Botox) can be injected in minute doses into the affected muscle. This toxin, produced by certain bacteria, paralyses muscle fibres and causes the injected muscle fibres to relax and spasticity to lessen. The effects last a couple of months before requiring additional injection again.

In the most severely affected cases that are unresponsive to physiotherapy, splints and medical treatment referral for cutting off the effected muscle tendons may be required.

General Advice for Spasticity

- Be aware of the signs of it and mention it to the treating team.
- Be aware of the side effects of any particular medications for spasticity.
- If your loved one is prescribed splints, try and encourage them to wear them.

SENSORY NEGLECT SYNDROMES

A less common set of symptoms that may be seen in brain injury is that of sensory neglect. This is associated with damage to the parietal lobe in particular and is most often seen in severe brain injuries. Neglect is associated with an individual being less aware or concerned about one side of their body. They will tend to ignore objects located on that side and in extreme versions of it will only eat food on the unaffected side of the plate or be unable to complete a clock drawing on the affected side. On a practical level, neglect can lead to the individual tending to accidentally bump the neglected side of their body. They may have difficulty walking through doors without hitting the affected side. Crossing the road can be a challenge as they may tend to avoid looking to the affected side. Occupational therapists will have a role in the assessment of the extent of the symptoms and how to manage and compensate for them.

APRAXIAS

Individuals with preserved power on one side may still be unable to perform meaningful tasks with that limb due to a condition called apraxia which is associated with damage to the parietal lobe, the part of the brain which has a role in spatial awareness and co-ordinating information related to the senses. This is usually diagnosed by occupational therapists when they notice that an affected limb may have power but not have function and the individual mightn't be able to use a hairbrush or other tools in that hand. Occupational therapists will usually work with the affected individual and try and come up with strategies to compensate.

HORMONAL PROBLEMS AFTER A BRAIN INJURY

Hormones are chemical messengers within the body; examples include thyroxine, oestrogen, and testosterone. They are produced by endocrine glands. The thyroid, pancreas, testicles, and ovaries are all examples of glands. Hormone production and release is controlled from the pituitary gland which manages the whole system. The pituitary produces a variety of hormones that stimulate the glands outside the brain to release hormones. It is pea sized and lies partly outside the brain, just beneath the brain in a small cave-like indentation in the skull and is linked to the hypothalamus via a narrow stalk. One of the problems with the location of the pituitary deep within the base of the skull means that it is very sensitive to head injuries and can be damaged by blows to the head and traumatic brain injury.

One of the most common hormone abnormalities seen after a brain injury is called SIADH (syndrome of inappropriate ADH secretion). Anti-diuretic hormone (ADH) is produced by the hypothalamus and functions to cause the kidneys to reabsorb as much water as possible to prevent dehydration and ensure that the concentration of water in the body is at a healthy level. After a brain injury, especially if the base of the skull or facial bones are damaged, too much ADH may be released. As a result more and more water is reabsorbed into the kidneys and the concentration of fluids within the body gets more dilute leading to a low amount of sodium in the blood stream. The medical term for low sodium is hyponatraemia and is associated with a variety of symptoms including nausea, weakness, tiredness, confusion and in worst cases seizures, coma or even death. Treatment usually involves restricting the amount of water the patient consumes. In most cases after a brain injury SIADH resolves with time and is only temporary.

Damage to the pituitary gland can cause hypopituitarism which occurs when production of one or more hormones is reduced, or panhypopituitarism which occurs when production of *all* pituitary hormones is reduced. The signs of underactive hormone production are variable depending on the hormones affected. However, symptoms include fatigue, weakness or reduced sex drive. If the male or female hormone production is affected symptoms such as lack of periods can be seen in women, or reduced libido, erections or beard growth in men. Hormonal problems often present with very vague symptoms and can very easily be missed.

HYDROCEPHALUS

The brain has a number of mechanisms and support structures to protect itself. Obviously, a hard, tough outer skull is one of these. However, a less obvious means of protection is cerebrospinal fluid (CSF) which, as we discussed in earlier chapters, is a clear fluid that surrounds the brain within the skull and can act as a sort of shock absorber. The 150 mls of CSF is produced deep within the brain and is pooled in spaces called ventricles and passes into other small spaces deep within the brain through very small spaces before exiting to bathe the surface of the brain before being re-absorbed. Whilst only 150 mls are present at any one time in the brain, around 500 mls are produced daily. This also helps in removing some waste from the brain, however the downside is that if there is a blockage within the system trouble can occur quickly due to a build-up of fluid. The fact that the skull is solid means that the pressure builds up and puts pressure on the brain itself causing it to be compressed. The small size of gaps within the pathway of the CSF in the brain means that a blockage within the system can develop. That build up is called hydrocephalus, which literally means water on the brain.

Whilst a lot of cases of hydrocephalus occur as a result of birth defects it can easily develop later in life as a result of blockages due to bleeds, tumours or trauma. The increased pressure within the brain produces symptoms, the most common being headache, vomiting, and increased confusion or drowsiness. However, the symptoms can often be very vague and difficult to immediately identify. Untreated hydrocephalus can lead to serious cognitive and neurological disabilities and can, at its extreme, cause death. The investigation of choice to out rule hydrocephalus is a brain scan – either CT brain or MRI brain.

Severe hydrocephalus is a neurosurgical emergency and is treated through inserting a tube (or shunt) into the brain to drain the fluid, which is connected to an external drain that collects the fluid. Due to risks of serious infection, an external drain is only a short-term measure. Individuals requiring longer term shunts will have a small tube inserted which runs from the brain to the inside of the abdomen where the drained CSF is reabsorbed by the body. These longer-term drains have valves and mechanisms to regulate pressure within the brain, preventing too much fluid being removed, preventing the individual getting a distressing low-pressure headache.

DEMENTIAS

Dementia is a neurological condition associated with progressive cognitive decline. Alzheimer's disease is the most common type of dementia and is associated with progressive deterioration in short-term memory over time. It is beyond doubt that individuals such as boxers who suffer repeated knocks to the head regularly and over many years are at a higher risk of dementia. However, it's less clear whether a single brain injury is associated with higher risks of dementia. Certainly, some post-mortem studies of the brains of individuals who have suffered an ABI have shown the same cellular changes as individuals with a dementia.

Dementias generally develop very gradually over time and in themselves can be a risk factor for falls and consequent brain injuries. For example, an elderly individual with dementia may wander at night and fall and suffer a brain injury. The dementia which was present may therefore only be noticed after the head injury.

HEADACHES AFTER A BRAIN INJURY

Headaches are a common occurrence after any brain injury. They can occur for a variety of reasons and are seen in individuals with mild, moderate and severe brain injuries. One thing that isn't a cause of the headaches is the direct damage to the brain itself. The brain doesn't have pain receptors that detect damage. Indeed, some forms of brain surgery for epilepsy can take place with the individual awake whilst the neurosurgeon dissects parts of the brain away. Instead, headache after a brain injury is either due to damage to nerves outside the brain that serve the head and neck or due to blood vessels. The sudden acceleration and deceleration forces seen in traumatic brain injuries may cause damage to some of the spinal nerves that emerge from the spine in the neck and that partly innervate the scalp. Stress, immobilisation, medications and other factors may well increase headache symptoms in the post-recovery period.

One important form of a headache that is very commonly seen after a brain injury is medication overuse or analgesic overuse headache. These headaches are associated with a dull pain that briefly reduces when the individual takes paracetamol or other painkillers only to return when the effect of the drug wears off. The individual then takes more paracetamol and gets into a yo-yo like cycle. Studies suggest that taking painkillers may over sensitise the body and actually increase the sensation of pain. Treatment for an analgesic overuse headache involves stopping taking paracetamol or painkillers and only taking the painkiller if the pain is intolerable. A small dose of amitriptyline, a sedative antidepressant is often prescribed for night-time in the hope of desensitising the pain and assisting sleep. Amitriptyline can, however, worsen memory as well as causing symptoms like dry mouth and urinary problems, so it's best to take lower doses initially at least.

Tension headaches are the most common type of headache and consist of a tight band-like feeling across the head similar to having a vice-grip squeezing head. It used to be thought that tension headaches were due to muscle spasm; however, research has shown that's not the case, though gentle massage of the head can help to reduce the pain.

Migraine is a special form of headache associated with a throbbing-like pain – usually behind the eye on one side of the head. In the classical form, it is associated with an aura consisting of a reduction of the visual field or other visual symptoms immediately before the onset of the pain. The pain itself is associated with photophobia, meaning that bright lights irritate the individual, as do loud noises or strong smells. The individual may feel irritable and the symptoms usually respond well to spending time in a darkened and quiet room and sleeping. Regular migraines may require use of tablets to prevent the onset.

Headaches are very commonly experienced after brain haemorrhages, particularly sub-arachnoid bleeds. These usually respond to low-dose painkillers but frequently the individual can become fearful that it is evidence of another bleed and may get into a cycle of repeated presentations to casualty.

Whilst the vast majority of headaches after a brain injury are innocent and not serious, a minority can be suggestive of problems. The red flag signs that should lead the individual to seek medical help include:

- Sudden onset and severe headache which reaches maximum severity within 5 minutes, like a clap of thunder
- a new onset headache in over 50-year-olds
- persistent headache which is worsening
- headache associated with neurological signs, for example reduced power in one limb
- associated with neck stiffness
- associated with a seizure

- associated with confusion, vomiting or worsened by lying down

If in any doubt seek medical help, especially if the headache is new onset, severe and new in character.

General Advice for Headaches

- Avoid taking paracetamol or pain killers too regularly.
- Avoid caffeine and drink plenty of fluids if the headache is a migraine.
- Meditation and mindfulness are effective for tension headaches and migraines.
- Acupuncture can also have a role in helping migraines[11] and tension headaches.[12]
- Vitamin B and magnesium may also be beneficial in preventing migraines.

CSF LEAK/CSF RHINORRHEA

Very occasionally an individual who has suffered a brain injury may report experiencing a continual drip of a clear colourless fluid from the nose. This drip may commence straight after the brain injury or sometime later. The drip may also come and go. The individual will complain of a particular form of headache that is worse when sitting or standing up and resolves when lying down. It becomes worse as the day progresses. They may also report tasting a salty fluid dripping into their throat and it may be associated with nausea, vomiting, neck stiffness or other neurological symptoms.

Symptoms of this headache need to be reported to doctors and investigated. Whilst it is fortunately a relatively rare phenomenon, it can be serious and life threatening. The headache is due to a small tear

---

[11] Linde K, Allais G, Brinkhaus B, et al. Acupuncture for the prevention of episodic migraine. *Cochrane Database Syst Rev*. 2016;2016(6):CD001218.
[12] Linde K, Allais G, Brinkhaus B, et al. Acupuncture for the prevention of tension-type headache. *Cochrane Database Syst Rev*. 2016;4:CD007587.

in the meninges and as a result, the CSF in the subarachnoid space drips through and eventually exits out of the nose or throat. Bacteria can get into the brain via the tear and lead to development of potentially life-threatening bacterial meningitis.

The doctor will take a sample of the fluid and send it to a laboratory for testing to confirm that it is indeed CSF. If it's confirmed that there is a leak, the individual will need to be seen by an ear, nose and throat doctor (ENT) who will investigate further and try and find the source of the tear and plug it in surgery.

CHAPTER TWELVE

Mental Health Problems After A Brain Injury

DEPRESSION AND ABI

Depression is perhaps one of the most overused and abused of words in the English language. It can mean very different things to different people and different doctors. It can range in severity from mild/minor 'blues' where somebody feels upset about things to very severe clinical depression where the individual takes to their bed and is unable to function. From a medical perspective, clinical or major depression is a condition associated with low mood and a host of other physical symptoms including insomnia, reduced appetite, reduced enjoyment, and reduced energy. Clinical depression usually is highly inheritable and individuals with the condition often have relatives who also suffer from it. Whilst stresses in life may precipitate a relapse of depression, this is not always the case and clinical depression often strikes for no apparent reason at all.

Just because an individual reports low mood doesn't make them clinically depressed. We live in an age that unfortunately attempts to medicalise all human experience. Adjustment disorders, grief reactions, dysthymia or personality disorders are all labels that can be used to reduce the experience of human suffering into a neat tick-box classified diagnosis for low mood. The most vital difference between clinical depression and these other causes of low mood is that antidepressant medications may be beneficial in clinical depression, whereas the likelihood of them being of use in the other states is far less likely. Talking therapies may offer a better alternative in such cases.

Symptoms of low mood are very common after a brain injury. Some studies suggest that up to two-thirds can have some degree of depressive symptoms after a brain injury. This fact is hardly surprising given the physical, emotional, and social factors that come into play after a brain injury.

Causes of Depression After a Brain Injury

Any brain injury – be it mild, moderate or severe – is a lot to deal with emotionally. Dealing with the physical losses such as memory problems, the problems with speech, challenges with walking or using one's hands and the frustration at not being as independent can all take a serious toll on anyone's emotional well-being. Loss of independence is never easy at any age but after a brain injury that loss is sudden and unexpected. Along with the loss/reduction of independence can also be loss or, at the very least, prolonged absence from employment or from other roles that the individual fulfilled prior to their injury. These losses have to be grieved by the individual and the duration of grief varies from individual to individual. In some, this mourning can take many years. Other emotional factors can also predispose the individual to depressive symptoms, particularly previous pre-injury stresses or poor ways with coping with adversities.

The brain is physically altered during an injury from bleeds, bruising and the sudden deceleration motions that can damage the microscopic neurons. Damaged brain cells don't work quite as well and also suffer from inflammatory responses that affects the delicate chemistry of the brain and easily lead to depression. In addition, the brain itself isn't the only part of the body often damaged after an accident. The individual may have other bones broken and sustained additional injuries causing pain, which itself is associated with depression. Some of the medications given in hospital, particularly steroids, or some anti-epileptic medications can also contribute to the risk of depression.

Brain injuries are also associated with lots of social changes which can be a cause of depression. One of the big social changes associated with loss of a job is the reduction in income and resulting changes to lifestyle. For many of us, our social life may revolve around work and loss of, or prolonged absence from, work can lead to loneliness. In many cases, legal proceedings such as compensation claims or criminal proceedings follow brain injuries. These are stressful for the individual and family members and unfortunately the legal system with its slow and adversarial manner doesn't make things any easier.

Symptoms of Depression

One of the challenges of diagnosing depression after a brain injury is that many of the physical symptoms seen in depression can also be present when an individual is affected with pain or cognitive problems.

The most important symptom of depression is a persistent low mood which remains low even when nice things, such as the visit of a family member, occurs. Things that the individual used to enjoy or take pleasure from no longer interest them and they constantly feel down. They feel miserable all the time. Some will notice that they feel particularly depressed in the morning time and that their mood lifts a little as the day progresses. The individual can become less sociable and want to be left alone and can also feel irritable. They can become preoccupied with things that they did in the past and can express guilt about their previous actions. They may ruminate about their accident or the cause of their brain injury.

In some, the mood can drop to the level that the individual expresses the wish that they didn't survive the accident or trauma that led to the injury. Family members need to be aware that risk of suicide is significantly higher in those who have sustained a brain injury and need to realise that some survivors of a brain injury can become suicidal. If the individual affected by brain injury expresses thoughts of harming themselves, then family members need to seek medical or psychiatric help and minimise access to medications or other means that could be used for suicide.

Diagnosing depression after a brain injury isn't simple – a number of symptoms usually associated with depression are commonly experienced after a brain injury, regardless of whether the individual is depressed or not. Low energy and fatigue are commonly seen after a brain injury, but are also seen in depression. Sleep problems also commonly occur. If the individual is depressed, however, they will be more likely to complain of wakening up earlier than normal in the morning and not being able to get back to sleep even though they still feel tired and want to sleep. They will generally experience a fitful and poor-quality sleep and won't feel refreshed after sleeping. Appetite will also be reduced and foods that they used to enjoy will be pushed to the side and not eaten. Weight loss can result, though in some cases the opposite may happen and the individual may eat additional comfort foods and gain weight. However, loss of appetite after a brain injury is seen if the individual has also lost their sense of smell and taste. Another very common cause of reduced appetite is related to the fact that hospital food can be repetitive and unappealing. In such cases it is worth checking whether take-away or home-cooked food might be preferred by the individual. Family members should ask nursing staff or speech and language therapists for advice on suitability of a particular food, given risk of choking in some after a brain injury.

Tearfulness is also frequently seen after a brain injury and can be associated with damage to parts of the brain that act like an emotional brake and stop all of us from crying when we hear sad things. Therefore, someone with a brain injury can be extremely weepy and tearful and not actually be depressed.

Similarly, some survivors with brain injury can appear very apathetic due to damage to the frontal lobes. To all intents and purpose they may appear depressed but their symptoms are due to the brain damage itself (see the case report titled "apathy" in chapter thirteen).

TREATMENT OF DEPRESSION

The treatment of depression depends on its severity and cause. The most important first step is proper diagnosis and out ruling other causes such as undertreated pain, infection or other physical sources. Milder cases of depression respond well to psychological treatments such as CBT, mindfulness, relaxation training or counselling.

Talking Therapies

Counselling or a regular listening ear is nearly always worthwhile. The world after a brain injury can be a scary place and discussing those fears and uncertainties can be useful. This doesn't have to be done just with a trained counsellor – many survivors of ABI get a lot of support from meeting other survivors, and attending local brain injury charity events can be particularly useful. Similarly, the banter between inpatients at rehabilitation facilities can be also very therapeutic. However, it's frequently easier for the individual to speak with a trained professional rather than a family member and discuss some of their innermost fears and worries after their brain injury, particularly when the whole family is distressed

CBT is a specific form of a talking therapy that can be used in depression. It consists of a specified number of sessions with a therapist who encourages the individual to examine the relationship between negative thoughts, feelings and behaviours. CBT has a very different philosophy from traditional counselling or psychotherapy. Firstly, it is very 'here and now' based, meaning that whilst issues from the past may be discussed, the primary focus is on dealing with problems from the present. Secondly, it is time limited and courses of CBT are generally shorter than traditional psychotherapy. Thirdly, it is a very active form of therapy and the therapist may give the individual homework to do and actively challenge some of the individual's thoughts rather than traditional psychotherapy or counselling where the individual is allowed to ventilate their thoughts. CBT sessions are highly structured.

The philosophy behind CBT is that our thoughts and our behaviours affect how we feel. Thinking about certain negative thoughts can make you feel low, upset and hopeless (feelings) and mean that you become reluctant to talk with family or friends (behaviours). The therapist may ask the individual to examine how realistic some of these thoughts or beliefs are and challenge them through completing experiments. CBT is widely available in the UK through the Improving Access to Psychological Therapies (IAPT) services. In addition, CBT is also available online, though online CBT is probably more suitable for those who have suffered milder brain injuries.

Mindfulness is a form of therapy that uses aspects of Eastern philosophy and meditation practices to deal with worries and low moods. The goal of it is to facilitate acceptance of distressing thoughts and to allow them to float away, using consciousness of one's breathing and other sensations to live in the present rather than be preoccupied with thoughts about the past or future. This treatment is especially useful for chronic pain symptoms and a number of books are available with CDs containing mindfulness exercises.

Relaxation training is similar to mindfulness in that it uses breathing exercises or imagery to feel more relaxed. It lacks the philosophical depth of mindfulness but can also be used through CDs or MP3s and is particularly useful in anxiety conditions.

Exploratory psychotherapy is used less often but still has its place. It is particularly useful in individuals that have pre-brain injury personality problems and a history of chronic low self-esteem, chronic feelings of emptiness and serious traumas in their past for whom short-term counselling would be not enough. It takes the form of one-to-one work with a professional psychotherapist who explores the association between current feelings and past experiences in a supportive environment over a prolonged period of time.

Social Therapy

Group therapy is a psychological treatment which isn't widely available outside the voluntary sector but can be of enormous benefit – particularly for those with milder symptoms. The therapy can be led by either a psychologist or trained facilitator. It takes the form of ABI survivors meeting together and discussing their frustrations and lives on a weekly basis. The therapy is useful in that it allows participants to receive and offer support to each other and also educates them that they are not alone in their difficulties. It can also create a sense of meaning and structure in the lives of those after a brain injury and reduce the sense of isolation that in itself can cause depression.

Medication

Antidepressant medication comes in many shapes and sizes. It is especially useful when the depression or anxiety is severe and affecting the individual on a daily basis. Despite what is believed among the general public, antidepressants are not addictive. Neither are they associated with increased risk of suicide. Studies have found that in general they reduced rates of self-harm, though still should be used with a lot of caution in those under eighteen years old. A third misconception is that it can cause someone to feel like a 'zombie'. Some antidepressants certainly can help sleep and as a side effect can give hangover-like symptoms but these are generally short-lived.

Serotonin specific reuptake inhibitors (SSRIs) are a particular class of antidepressants that boost levels of serotonin, a chemical in the brain that is thought to be reduced in depression and anxiety. There are many different types including fluoxetine (of which Prozac™ is a brand), citalopram (of which Cipramil™ is a brand), sertraline (of which Lustral™ is a brand) and paroxetine (of which Seroxat™ is a brand). The main side effect associated with them is nausea, which can be a problem especially for a couple of weeks after starting the tablets. The best way of preventing nausea is to take the medication along with food and to be aware that this side effect reduces as the body gets used to the tablet. This class of medications has been used safely for many years and citalopram in particular interacts with very few other medications and is also available in liquid form.

Serotonin and noradrenaline reuptake inhibitors (SNRIs) are another class of antidepressants. Examples of SNRIs include venlafaxine (or Effexor™) or duloxetine (or Cymbalta™). Duloxetine is also licenced for and widely used in those with chronic pain.

Mirtazepine (of which Zispin™ is a brand) is a specific form of antidepressant that also helps with sleep, and so should be taken at night-time. However, it can be associated with weight gain, which can be an advantage particularly in individuals who have a very low appetite.

Tricyclic antidepressants are an older group of antidepressants. They are used less often now due to their side effects, due to the fact that they are more lethal if taken in an overdose, and because they also interact with other medications. One type, amitriptyline, is still widely used in cases of chronic pain, albeit at a low dose.

Antidepressants generally will take between a fortnight and three weeks to work. They are started at a low dose and this may need to be increased to a higher dose to be effective.

Recent research suggests that an additional benefit of antidepressants is that they appear to have a role in increasing neuroplasticity and enhance the development of new connections between neurons to compensate for the brain damage.

Advice for Family Members on Dealing with Depressive Problems:

- Be aware of the risk of depression developing after a brain injury and if in doubt seek advice from the treating team or general practitioner.
- Don't ignore it. Presence of depression is associated with poorer prognosis and outcome, and causes distress for families and carers. Improved mental health is associated with better outcome. Depression itself, particularly chronic depression, is toxic and damaging to the brain.
- Don't offer silly platitudes to someone like 'it will be all right' or 'pull yourself together'. This will just cause them to be less confiding.
- Do encourage and remind them to take antidepressant medications if they are prescribed by their doctors.
- Be aware of the higher risks of suicide in individuals after a brain injury, whether they are depressed or not. An individual expressing suicidal thoughts or thoughts that life isn't worth living isn't looking for attention and needs to be listened to, and care and advice needs to be sought from professions in such circumstances.

In hospital settings inform staff if you are concerned about a loved one's mood or risk of self-harm. In the community bring them to their GP or in cases of emergency, the local casualty department.

- Encourage a good diet and try and avoid them getting into a pattern of skipping meals or subsisting on a tea and toast diet. If they are deficient in vitamins and minerals then mood will remain low.

- Try and encourage them to go out and do some mild exercise, like walking if they are able to. It does boost the energy and mood.

Advice for Individuals Dealing with Depressive Problems:

- Seek help if you believe you are depressed. If everybody who felt depressed was able to deal with it alone then there wouldn't be need for so many support services out there. Seeking help isn't weakness. Talking about how you are feeling to family, friends, or professionals can save your life.

- Stop stigmatising yourself — it's not your fault if you feel depressed. You're not overly sensitive, unstable, mad, lost or any of the other adjectives you think you are.

- Far more people care for you and love you than you realise. Avoiding them and hiding away from them just makes you feel worse.

- Do try and get involved in activities that give you pleasure and that improve your mood, even if only for a short while.

- Physical activity can help improve mood — try and be as active as you're able to be.

- Avoid alcohol or drugs, they will just make you feel worse the next day.

- Try and eat a healthy three meals per day even if you don't feel hungry.

- If you're prescribed antidepressants, take them regularly. They won't help your mood improve if you take them haphazardly.

CASE HISTORY: DEPRESSION AFTER A BRAIN INJURY?

Amy was a 28-year-old mother of two children. She sustained a severe brain injury and fractured a number of ribs when she fell down the stairs. She suffered some bruising to the brain, as well as a very small bleed. However, she did not require any surgical intervention and was discharged from hospital fairly quickly.

On returning home, her family noticed that she was far quieter in herself, and less active than she used to be. The family also wondered if she was depressed, since she would occasionally be tearful if she had seen something sad on the television. She was sleeping poorly at night-time, but this was due to her ribs causing a lot of pain. She was also very tired a lot of the time and found having her children in the house very tiring. When asked if she was depressed, she denied this and just said that she was a bit fed up with her current situation. She continued to enjoy playing with her children and meeting friends, though her tiredness meant that she didn't get to do this as often as she'd like. She denied any thoughts that life was not worth living, and she was keen to get back to her old lifestyle, but felt very tired a lot of the time.

This is not an uncommon case after a brain injury. Amy's family, who clearly cared greatly for her, were worried that she was depressed. They noted that she was quieter, more tearful, and less active. It is easy to think that the constellation of such symptoms automatically meant depression. However, in Amy's case, she continued to enjoy being with her family. She reported poor sleep but this was due to the physical pain. She was also a lot less motivated, but then again, she had lots of problems due to fatigue. Her tearfulness may well have been related to her frontal lobe bruising or due to the fact that she felt grateful to be back with her family again. The fact that she denied feeling depressed is an important one, as is her clear desire to get back to being independent and active again. Overall, there was no real evidence that she was depressed. If her tearfulness was embarrassing for her, then she could be put on a low dose of an antidepressant to stop it. However, in cases such as Amy's, it's best to adopt a 'wait and see' approach. If her mood remained low even after her pain issues settled, then it might be worthwhile reviewing to see if she is indeed depressed.

ANXIETY AFTER AN ACQUIRED BRAIN INJURY

Anxiety is frequently a bigger issue after a mild ABI than a severe ABI. A number of types of anxiety can develop after an ABI and can range greatly in severity.

PANIC ATTACKS

A panic attack is the name given to episodes of intense anxiety. It is associated with a number of physical and emotional symptoms.

The physical symptoms experienced include:
• dry mouth
• palpations or fast beating of the heart
• fast and shallow breathing
• shaky hands
• a feeling of butterflies in the tummy
• and feelings of wanting to vomit

At the same time as these bodily sensations, the individual will experience the feeling of intense fear and worry that they are going to die or that something terrible is going to happen. This will often be associated with a desire to escape to a place of safety or to get away from a crowded environment.

The panic attacks themselves last only up to five minutes but may occur in clusters one after another or last until the perceived threat is gone or the individual is in a safe place. After the panic attack, the individual will feel tired, upset, drained and down. They may ruminate and think over and over about the panic attack and how they reacted or didn't react during it or what they said or didn't say. They'll generally berate themselves and feel embarrassed, inept and silly and tend to blame themselves. One of the tendencies associated with panic attacks is to associate it with whatever they were doing or wherever they were when it happened. Avoidance can become a key problem and the individual may avoid being in that place or circumstance again. With time, the number of places they'll avoid becomes more and more so that they become increasingly housebound and will not go out alone. In some respects, the true problem with panic attacks doesn't lie in the fact that they happen, it lies in the individual's response to them and the resulting avoidance.

GENERALISED ANXIETY

Associated with panic attacks is generalised anxiety which is present most of the time. Generalised anxiety disorder is basically a medical term for feeling scared, afraid, tense and fearful all of the time or a lot of the time, particularly in places or situations out of the ordinary or away from home. The individual will experience the same physical symptoms of tremors, sweating, increased heart rate, and stomach butterflies but not to the same crippling extent seen in panic attacks. However, they will feel afraid all or a lot of the time. They may also report anticipatory anxiety and will feel more scared before they have to go somewhere or attend a particular appointment. As a result of the anticipatory anxiety, they may display a tendency to avoid particular social situations where their anxiety is worse. Even if they do attend, there can be a tendency to feel uncomfortable and find it difficult to relax and be keen to get away. They may feel hypervigilant and find themselves constantly looking over their shoulders and as a result will feel restless and have poor concentration. They also may startle easily and have a tendency to react or jump with loud noises. They'll report feeling on edge all the time and if they are especially distressed, they may get a sensation that things are unreal or a feeling that they are losing control and going to pass out.

In the case of brain injury, an individual can become panicky and anxious in social situations, particularly if they feel that others are looking at a disability or scar that they might have. Circumstances similar to those associated with the cause of the brain injury can also lead to an increased level of fear and avoidance. An example of this might be getting anxious when getting into a car when the brain injury occurred as a result of a car crash.

POST-TRAUMATIC STRESS DISORDER

Post-traumatic stress disorder (PTSD), previously called shell shock, is an extreme form of an anxiety disorder that can develop after a trauma and is associated with reliving a trauma over and over again. The different kinds of traumas that can produce PTSD are generally life threatening and very distressing.

In moderate to severe brain injury, the survivor will have no recollection of the trauma due to amnesia. As already mentioned in Chapter one, retrograde amnesia may be so bad that the individual will have no recollection of the day or even days before the accident. It used to be believed that people with severe brain injury could not experience PTSD because of this amnesia and so could not have flashbacks. However, this is likely incorrect since even those with a severe brain injury may recall fragments of a trauma and many will fill in the memories based on what they hear from family members and others.

PTSD is associated with a number of symptoms, including flashbacks, where the individual experiences intense images, sounds or smells reminiscent of the traumatic event. These flashbacks are distressing and cause the individual to feel like they are reliving the trauma again. In addition, the individual will be avoidant of things or reminders associated with the trauma. For example, they may avoid travelling by car or passing where the accident took place. Such avoidant behaviours can be very subtle and the individual may try to rationalise them. The avoidance is often associated with a sense of shame and frequently will not be admitted to. The individual may report distressing nightmares involving the trauma. They may deliberately avoid talking about the trauma and become irritable if anyone tries to discuss it. As a result, they can become distant from relatives and friends. When challenged on the trauma, they may have reduced abilities to remember the sequence of events or important aspects of what happened through blocking the memories out. They will show signs of hypervigilance or constantly looking over their shoulder, startling easily or being jumpy in response to sudden noises, being irritable, and sleeping lightly and wakening if there is any noise at all.

TREATMENT OF ANXIETY DISORDERS

In the past, many forms of anxiety were treated with tranquilisers such as diazepam. The problem with these medications is that they are very addictive and after a while lose their efficacy so that a higher dose needs to be taken. Doctors are therefore now very reluctant to prescribe these tablets and will only do so for short periods of time. Antidepressant medications, however, are often used for anxiety as they have the advantage of not being addictive and are also useful for co-morbid depressive symptoms that are frequently associated with anxiety disorders. In the case of PTSD, the dose of the antidepressant used needs to be higher. Other medications that are used to help treat anxiety include pregabalin, which is licenced for use in generalised anxiety disorder. This drug, which was originally developed to be used as an anti-epileptic medication, is also used in management of pain and can aid with sleep. Increasingly, there are concerns that this medication may be addictive and it has recently been reclassified as a controlled drug. A blood pressure tablet called propranolol is also occasionally used in the treatment of anxiety as it lowers the heart rate. Though it should be used with caution in individuals with asthma. Propranolol can also cause low blood pressure and unsteadiness on standing up suddenly.

Psychological therapies can also be helpful in the treatment of anxiety and are particularly useful with milder forms. In the case of PTSD, a number of specific psychological interventions exist. Graded desensitisation is a behavioural intervention that sometimes forms part of a cognitive behavioural approach. It relies on the fact that we can all overcome fears and phobias by breaking the problem into small steps. As a therapeutic approach, it is particularly useful in managing avoidance or specific phobias related to the trauma. For example, in the case of someone who is afraid of being in a car after a road collision, the therapy can start by getting the individual to look at pictures of cars and making them focus on the picture until their anxiety reduces. The therapist can in subsequent sessions bring the individual to a stationary car and have them remain beside it until their anxiety reduces. Over time, this can progress to sessions involving sitting in a stationary car, sitting in a car with the engine on and then being a passenger in a moving car. The therapy relies on the fact than an individual gradually gets used to or desensitises to a trauma.

EMDR or eye movement desensitisation is a specific form of psychotherapy where the individual relives the trauma during a therapy session whilst moving their eyes in particular pattern, usually in time to a metronome. Over a number of sessions, the individual gets less distressed at thinking about and reliving the trauma in their mind.

CBT is particularly useful in anxiety disorders after a milder brain injury. Similar to CBT in depression, the therapy is one-to-one and will take the form of initially using a diary to become aware of the situations that predispose to anxious feelings and examining with the therapist the thoughts and behaviours that occur as a result. The link between anxious thoughts, behaviours and feelings is broken through use of experiments and through questioning the validity of some of those behaviours. The therapist often uses graded desensitisation and exercises to help in these situations. Graded exposure and desensitisation consist of creating a hierarchy of fears, from the least anxiety provoking to the greatest. The therapist and the individual then start to overcome the least anxiety-provoking situations and progress to the more anxiety-provoking ones.

Advice for Family Members on Dealing with Anxiety Problems:

- Awareness and early identification are key. If you notice that loved ones have increasing issues with anxiety discuss it with the individual's doctors or treating team.

- Support: many individuals who develop anxiety can be very self-conscious and ashamed about it, particularly if they've presented a macho or tough appearance to the world before their injury. Family and friends can support their loved one in such cases by normalising any anxiety and not stigmatising them.

- Be sensitive when discussing the circumstances of the accident and be open to the fact that the loved one might find such discussions very distressing.

- Do not stigmatise or demean the individual for being anxious.

- Avoiding avoidance: Family and friends have a vitally important role in supporting their loved one at every stage of their recovery. However, there is a difference between support and enabling. One of the key features of anxiety is avoidance. In cases of significant avoidance, especially after they've been at home a while, the family needs to gently but actively encourage the individual to challenge their anxieties and avoidances one step at a time.

- Mindfulness and relaxation tapes are readily available and worth using.

- Gentle reassurance and a listening ear can be very helpful.

CASE HISTORY: ANXIETY AFTER A BRAIN INJURY

Andrew was a 45-year-old man who enjoyed football and going drinking with his friends. One night, on returning home from his local pub, he was set upon by a number of individuals. He was beaten up and sustained significant head injuries as well as injuries to the rest of his body.

He was in a coma for a number of weeks and on regaining consciousness he was confused for some time. Whilst he did not require neurosurgical intervention, he had a lot of bruising and bleeds to his brain. He also reported problems with short-term memory. His family noted that over a six-month period, as his physical symptoms improved, he reported increasing amounts of anxiety. They found that he was far more tearful and he also became far less sociable and would not leave the house alone.

He became very upset when anyone suggested going to visit his local public house. When asked, he admitted to having distressing nightmares about being attacked. He also found it particularly distressing when family members or friends spoke about the assault, or when they described how he looked after he was found.

As part of the police investigation, he ended up having to look at some CCTV footage of his assault and he found this particularly distressing, and started to think about it again and again. His general practitioner diagnosed him with post-traumatic stress disorder.

This is a rather textbook case of PTSD. In Andrews's case, the potential consequences of staying at home are potentially very serious for him. He could easily become housebound and his reduced levels of socialisation could lead to depression. Prompt diagnosis and treatment – both with medications in the form of higher dose antidepressant and psychological interventions – are essential.

CASE HISTORY: PANIC ATTACKS AFTER A BRAIN INJURY

Lorraine is a 48-year-old mother of four children. She lived an independent and active life until she had a brain haemorrhage as a result of an aneurysm. Due to the size of the bleed, she ended up requiring a craniotomy to remove the clot. She recovered reasonably well but continued to experience lots of problems with fatigue and headaches. She used to get quite stressed and anxious about the headaches, as she was afraid it was evidence of a further bleed.

So bad was her fear that she ended up going to casualty a number of times. Every time she would develop a headache, she would get very tremulous and start hyperventilating. She used to be afraid that she was going to die from another bleed.

After a brain haemorrhage, fears of having further bleeds are very common, particularly in individuals who have additional untreated smaller aneurysms. In Lorraine's case, she was reporting a great deal of anticipatory anxiety. She was also hypervigilant and constantly monitoring herself for symptoms. If she noted any twinges she immediately thought this was evidence of a further bleed. She then developed the full constellation of symptoms associated with a panic attack. It is often surprisingly difficult for many people to realise that the physical symptoms they are getting are due to panic. Like a wolf in sheep's clothing, anxiety can present in many different ways.

Lorraine required CBT which looked at the set of beliefs that she had. Her therapist noted that Lorraine now believed that the world was fundamentally dangerous and that she was going to die of another bleed. The therapist also managed to identify a set of behaviours she exhibited when she was panic stricken. Her therapy took the form of educating her about the nature of panic attacks and practical things she could do to reduce the anxiety. Her general practitioner also started her on an antidepressant medication to complement the therapy she was getting and reduce her overall anxiety. Whilst Lorraine initially didn't want to go on medication, she found that she remained very anxious and was unable to participate fully in CBT until she was started on a low dose of an antidepressant.

SUBSTANCE MISUSE AND BRAIN INJURY

Alcohol and drug addictions represent the final common pathway and end stages of often deep-seated demons. It's all too easy to simply blame the alcoholic or addict for their habit. It's all too easy to become overwhelmed with a sense of frustration at their dependence on whatever substance they feel they require to give their life meaning or anaesthetise their soul from the pain within. We live in a world that is full of pain for a variety of reasons and so many of those that we know and love are losing the fight with their own battles, often for the want of opening up and being truthful with themselves as well as those around them. Their behaviour can feel like a hurtful betrayal and be painful in so many ways, so it's hardly surprising that our ineffectual response is to nag and lecture.

Alcohol and drug abuse are both risk factors for getting a brain injury. Falls can result from being intoxicated, both through the physical clumsiness associated with taking too much alcohol or drugs and also through taking more risks and being less safety consciousness when drunk or intoxicated. Those who are drunk are also at a higher risk of being physically assaulted which can be a cause of the head injury. Being intoxicated at time of brain injury is associated with poorer outcome and longer time spent in hospital. In addition, the social consequences of alcoholism such as homelessness, limited social supports and financial problems all make it harder for someone with addiction problems to safely return to their home; many require longer-term residential care and support.

One of the great disappointments in providing rehabilitation to someone with previous addictions occurs if they relapse and start drinking or taking drugs again after the period of rehabilitation is over. The intense effort of the multidisciplinary team is instantly made null and void as a result of going back to addiction.

Sadly, studies have found that there is nothing unusual about individuals recommencing drinking in the aftermath of a brain injury. One study found that two years after a brain injury a quarter of those with a history of alcohol problems will be drinking at dangerously high levels and a further 15% will have fully fledged alcoholism. In short, over a third learn nothing from the physical and emotional trauma that they and their families have been through. Those at the highest risk of going back to drinking again include the young, males, those with a history of addiction and those with family history of addiction and alcoholism. Not surprisingly, therefore, substance misuse after a brain injury is associated with poorer outcome and higher risk of further brain injury.

Families need to be very aware of a relapse in drinking or drug taking, particularly in those with severe pre-brain injury addiction issues. They need to be quick to identify drink-seeking behaviour and point out the dangers associated with this. In cases of relapses they should encourage their loved one to get help from additions services. Family members need to actively stop denying that there is no problem and that their loved one is just 'good fun', 'great craic', 'likes a drink', 'is a party animal' and all the other empty excuses used to deny the presence of the problem.

The Signs of Alcohol/Drug Dependence Are Any of the Following:

- Primacy of drink/drug-seeking behaviour: getting access to alcohol/drugs comes first and is more important than job, friends, family etc.

- Subjective awareness of compulsion to drink/take drugs: the individual feels the need to drink alcohol or take drugs and craves it.

- Stereotyped pattern of drinking/drug taking. For example, drinking at the same time of the day in the same place.

- Narrowing of the repertoire: drinking the same types of alcohol e.g. beer, spirits etc. or same types of drugs

- Increasing tolerance: it takes larger amounts of alcohol to become intoxicated.

- Withdrawal symptoms including shaking, sweating, increased anxiety, feeling on edge or in extreme cases delirium tremens associated with confusion and occasionally seizures.

- Avoidance of withdrawal symptoms by drinking or taking drugs.

As a family member or even a friend it can be difficult to broach such issues and they can readily become chronic 'white elephants in the room' in relationships. However, there is help available for individuals with addictions and standing idly by and waiting for further brain injuries to occur is hardly conducive to honest or good relations. Einstein is **reputed** (probably erroneously) to have said that the definition of madness is repeating the same action and expecting different results. Using that train of thought, entering into a cycle of repeated brain injuries and further drug/alcohol taking is also pretty illogical and devoid of meaning.

GETTING HELP FOR MENTAL HEALTH PROBLEMS DUE TO BRAIN INJURY

One of the most frequent areas of frustration for individuals affected with brain injury and their families relates to getting help for the resulting psychiatric issues. For those with more severe problems, in the United Kingdom provision of neuropsychiatry and neuropsychology services is patchy and some community mental health teams can be reluctant to manage those with ABI or feel that they are unable to offer appropriate treatment. There is, alas, a considerable postcode lottery. Most regional neuroscience centres will have some access to neuropsychiatry; however, even these services are limited and consist of little more than the provision of outpatient clinic care.

For an unknown reason, community ABI teams often will have psychologists but lack psychiatrists. This causes considerable difficulties and means that those who are most vulnerable with co-morbid serious mental health and ABI issues lack the integrated care they so desperately require. The fact that a recent parliamentary report mentioned all areas related to brain injury and yet didn't mention mental health and ABI is further evidence of the level of stigma in this area.

Those who sustained their injury as a result of a criminal offence, road traffic collision or work-based accident and are pursuing compensation claims will have the additional benefit of access to private case management services and access to private neuropsychology and occasionally neuropsychiatry.

However, for the most part access to services will be limited to general practice and community mental health teams. Though far from ideal, this can be reasonably adequate for many patients with milder mental health challenges after an acquired brain injury.

In the United Kingdom at least, it may be possible for specialist additional input through individual funding requests which can be funded by the Clinical Commissioning Group (CCG) on application by a general practitioner or another specialist.

Psychological input is frequently limited to therapies associated with the Improvement Access to Psychological Therapies (IAPT) services.

In England, there are a limited number of inpatient rehabilitation facilities that offer services exclusively for those with cognitive and behavioural problems as a result of brain injury. Most of these are located within London but there are additional NHS centres in Liverpool, Stoke-on-Trent and Newcastle. These centres offer inpatient multidisciplinary input including neuropsychiatry, psychology, occupational therapy, physiotherapy and additional therapies for the affected individual and their family. Again, this can be funded through the CCG and an individual funding request.

However, the lack of neuropsychiatric services means that people with brain injuries can miss out on mental health care and fall between the cracks of services and society. Individuals with co-morbid mental health and brain injuries aren't good advocates for their health and frequently manage to alienate themselves owing to their behaviour. The common end point as a result can be homelessness, imprisonment, poverty, early death and suicide. It is hardly surprising then that many individuals who are homeless have had a brain injury at some point in their lives. Similarly, prisons are populated with prisoners who would be better off in rehabilitation settings.

And finally, rates of suicide in those after brain injuries are twice that of the general population in those with milder brain injuries and over 4 times than in more severe brain injuries.

CHAPTER THIRTEEN

Walking on Eggshells for Dr Jekyll: The Organic Personality Disorder

Who we are is one of the most fundamental of questions and one that has occupied many great thinkers over the years. In essence, we are the constellation of our experiences, our past, our circumstances, our temperament and our personality.

Personality is defined as the ingrained pattern of thinking, feeling and behaving. Whilst an individual's personality is greatly influenced by the sum of life experiences and genetics, the health or otherwise of their brain also plays an important role.

For weeks to months in the immediate aftermath of any brain injury, the survivor will be dazed, confused, emotional and plainly not themselves. This is perfectly natural and is as reflective of being in hospital and the physical injury as it is of any psychological or emotional reaction to the injury. A loved one in the immediate aftermath of the injury may display symptoms of post-traumatic amnesia (see chapter ten) or adjustment symptoms. Even if this isn't the case, the whole process of hospitalisation and rehabilitation is a myriad of daily frustrations and challenges. The inpatient environment itself is quite artificial and can create its own challenges of dependence and apathy. Any apparent changes in personality during these periods and in the immediate aftermath of discharge home is not unusual and alterations of behaviour should be expected, accepted (though don't have to be necessarily passively tolerated) and supported.

Any trauma or injury, whether it affects the brain or not, will alter the way that we look at the world and make us different people.

Whilst personality is often defined as being fixed, the whole process of living and growing as a person means that we all change with time in response to the slings and arrows of outrageous fortune which life throws at us.

Beyond the actual psychological reaction, the physical damage to the brain may be associated with significant changes in personality. This is particularly the case when the frontal lobes are damaged and especially in cases of severe brain injury. As already mentioned in the first chapter, the frontal lobe has a vital role in motivation, impulse control, organisation and social behaviours.

Severe frontal lobe injury can change a person's personality in a devastating manner with consequences for the individual themselves and for their family, friends and society as a whole.

PHINEAS GAGE: A LESSON FROM HISTORY

The true story of Phineas Gage is a cautionary one that is frequently mentioned in neurological textbooks or any books that discusses the frontal lobe and personality. Phineas was a young man from New Hampshire who worked as a foreman on the building of railways in the US in the 19th century. On one fateful day in 1860, he was laying an explosive charge in rural Vermont to clear rock so that railway track could be laid. The laying of the track involved stuffing the explosive into a hole in the rock with a long metal bar. Unfortunately, whilst stuffing the explosive, sparks prematurely detonated the explosive charge and in the ensuing explosion the bar was thrown at speed approximately 3 meters away. Phineas had his head placed just above the metal bar at the time of the explosion and the bar passed through his skull like a bullet. A huge gaping wound and hole was created from just under his left eye to the right side of his skull. He was left dazed but amazingly still alive and conscious at the side of the track, the metal bar a number of metres away. The doctor who treated him at the scene, noted that Phineas was able to talk and tell others what had happened to him before vomiting with half a cupful of brain tissue being forced through the wound in his head in the process. Remarkably, despite the absence of any antibiotics and the fact that the accident occurred in the era before medicine discovered the need for hygiene and asepsis, Phineas survived the injury. In the immediate aftermath the area around his head wound became very infected and he almost died. There is evidence that he was confused at times; at one point he left the boarding house where he was being treated without shoes and attempted to walk home in the snow.

Subsequent reports suggested that his personality dramatically changed, and that whilst prior to the injury he was hardworking, honest, and conscientious, after the injury he was described as being less responsible. A Mayo clinic neurosurgeon in a classic medical paper described him presenting after the injury with "a vainglorious tendency to show off his wound...inappropriate sexual behaviour, inability or refusal to hold a job, plus drinking, bragging, lying, gambling, brawling, bullying, and thievery".

A mythology around his story developed. Descriptions of his behaviour became more dramatic and striking in the retelling with time. In actual fact, he appears to have returned to doing some work on his parents' farm quite early. Unable to find work again on the railways, he made public appearances as a medical curiosity at Barnum's American Museum. He later worked in a stable before moving to Chile in South America for a time to drive stagecoaches, before ill health caused him to move to be with his mother and sister who had moved in the meantime to California. He developed severe epilepsy and died at the age of just 36.

Many historians question the actual historical accuracy of the description of his behaviour. One of the doctors who publicised his case was greatly interested in phrenology[13] and it appears may have embellished aspects of Phineas' tale to support his views on that pseudoscience. However, what is beyond doubt is the fact that some brain

---

[13] A pseudoscience popular in the 19th century that believed the location of indentations or bumps on the head was associated with various mental traits.

injuries are associated with devastating personality changes similar to those attributed to Gage.

SYMPTOMS OF FRONTAL LOBE DAMAGE

The frontal lobes are the last part of the brain to mature and don't fully develop until at least the early twenties. They have an important role in higher executive function, multitasking, decision-making and maintenance of social cues. The frontal lobe can be viewed in many ways as an organiser, as our conscience but best of all as a brake on our more malign desires and instincts.

After a serious injury to the frontal lobes, this safety valve on our behaviour can be strongly weakened, particularly in those that are young and whose brains haven't fully matured. The resultant behaviour is best compared to that of a nightmare teenager with similar levels of irresponsible behaviour and insight.

Impulsivity is a particular problem in frontal lobe injuries. The individual will act with no understanding of the consequences of their behaviour and will live for the moment and seek instant gratification, demanding their current desires and demands to be immediately fulfilled. That impulsivity may extend to many areas of life and degrees of impulsivity will vary greatly from person to person. Some will be impulsive in their purchases; they will instantly desire things that they don't need and will needlessly buy items of clothing, footwear, DVDs, technology, etc. with no regard for the cost or whether they actually require it. Purchases can frequently be left unopened, unused and amass in great quantity. That impulsivity can also extend to food; individuals will buy food, particularly takeaways, in quantities that they couldn't possibly consume or will attempt to consume huge quantities of food with the resultant gain in weight.

Consumption of alcohol or illicit drugs can also become an issue. This is a particular problem given the fact that alcohol and drugs will make the individual more disinhibited, worsening behavioural problems and creating a cycle of addiction. The individual can be impulsive in their decisions which are poorly thought-out and reckless with little consideration for their safety and the safety of others.

The ability to judge others and navigate social relationships can also be impaired, so that the individual may also start to mix with irresponsible or nasty people and as a result can get themselves into very dangerous situations with resultant risks for their safety and the safety of others. Relationships can be a particular problem area and the affected person will tend to attract potentially exploitative individuals who may exploit them for sex, drugs or money – this is particularly the case if the survivor is single or separated and has few social supports. The ultimate consequences of their behaviour are unlimited and can involve getting into trouble with the police, prison, pregnancy, sexually transmitted infections, homelessness, addiction, and further brain injuries.

Insight is a term used to describe an individual's understanding of their current circumstances and behaviours. Insight is invariably absent with severe frontal lobe damage. The individual will believe that they have no problem with their behaviour or cognition and that those around them are being unreasonable in trying to place limits on their behaviour and the fun they want to have. Presenting evidence to the contrary can be a frustrating and pointless exercise and one that will result in further denials, rages and accusations on the part of the individual towards their loved one. Managing and coping with such behaviours as a family member can involve a carefully negotiated tightrope between protecting their loved one and allowing them sufficient autonomy so that the resultant rages are bearable.

Whilst it can be possible to live with the impulsivity, immaturity, aggression and self-centeredness associated with personality change, the most upsetting aspect of the new personality can be the ultimate absence of any empathy at its core in extreme cases. Other people, including loved ones, are viewed as mere objects to be used and abused as means of fulfilling the individual's fleeting whim. More than any other change after a severe brain injury, it is the absence of empathy that can cause intense frustration and produce breakdowns in relationships. The absence of insight and empathy on the part of the individual means that they will blame others for everything and lack the sensitivity in their relations with others.

The frontal lobes have an important role in deferring our immediate and most primitive desires in terms of anger, aggression, sexual and destruction. They can be best realised as a backstop on our base desires. One part of behaviour that is affected after a brain injury is the ability we have to cope with annoyance. In all of our daily existence, we encounter annoyances and frustrations, be it from others, ourselves or the world in general. That ability to cope with those frustrations is affected greatly after a frontal lobe injury. Instead of biting our tongue and letting things pass, the individual with a frontal lobe injury will react intensely to frustration of any kind, be it trivial or significant. That response can be dramatic and explosive with anger directed towards objects, the individual themselves or others.

Direction of anger and aggression towards objects can take the form of slamming doors, stamping and kicking objects or throwing and breaking objects. Direction of anger and frustration towards the individual themselves can take the form of punching walls, scraping and cutting of their skin and actual self-harming behaviours. Direction of anger towards others can take the form of swearing, shouting and actual physical assaults or fighting.

Anger seen after a brain injury is quite different to the anger that can be seen in those with antisocial personality disorders. In the case of a brain injury, the anger is usually short-lived and explosive, departing as quickly as it occurs. The anger is unintended and the usual targets are family, friends and carers. Invariably the person with the brain injury feels intensely ashamed and guilty for what has happened after the episode of anger has abated. It usually occurs in response to a number of factors including being overly tired, too much noise and stimulation, being overloaded with information or questions and being challenged. Instinctively, those closest to the individual will learn to avoid certain topics or triggers, which can create its own difficulties and many families will describe a tense environment in the home of 'walking on eggshells' for fear of causing upset. Some families will never fully learn how to manage the situation and this can cause its own challenges and a pattern of repeated rows.

Triggers of Anger After a Brain Injury:

- fatigue
- over stimulation
- being in a loud and chaotic environment
- hunger
- too much caffeine
- alcohol or drugs
- being talked down to or perceived slights
- anxiety – particularly cues associated with initial brain injury
- depression
- lax boundaries and overindulgence by family members

One of the more frustrating aspects of the individual's personality seen after a severe frontal lobe injury is a tendency to see everything as a joke. The Germans term this 'witzelsucht' or silly prankish humour. The jokes invariably are repeated again and again and after a while the behaviour can become very grating. In the home environment, this can be quite amusing initially but becomes more of an issue outside of the home – especially if they develop a tendency to 'perform' when out. In addition to a tendency to be jocular and see the funny side of everything, the sense of diplomacy that is required in modern life may become absent, leading to a tendency to be brutally blunt to others, pointing out deficits and loudly laughing. In addition to causing embarrassment for family this can be potentially dangerous for the brain injury survivor as strangers subjected to the humorous comments may not appreciate that the individual has a brain injury and may react with violence.

Obsessional or repetitive behaviours may also be seen as part of frontal lobe damage. The individual may ask the same question again and again throughout the day or seek reassurance that something has been done already, such as repeatedly asking whether the front door was closed. The individual may become fixated on doing a particular task at a particular time and become distressed and annoyed if there are any barriers put in the way of their routine. Sometimes, it may be possible to replace unhelpful behaviours with a more acceptable one, for example substituting a very stereotyped form of drinking alcohol for a more acceptable one of cleaning the house in a particular pattern.

Very rarely, sexual disinhibition may also be a feature of a frontal lobe injury. The extent and severity of this behaviour can range from mild but inappropriate sexual innuendo-laden language or being more amorous with partners, to less common full scale serious sexual acts of masturbation or exhibitionism in public or groping or sexual assaults on others. A feature of sexualised behaviour seen after a brain injury that doesn't occur in non-brain injured offenders is the poorly planned and poorly thought-out nature of the acts. However, this is not to trivialise some of the potential for harm. The arrival of the internet has added an even higher level of risk for those with brain injuries. Young women with brain injuries in particular can end up in very vulnerable situations through online dating or adult sexual encounter sites.

The absence of insight into their cognitive problems means that younger individuals with brain injuries can have overly ambitious plans to meet partners and have their own families. This can become a particular issue when it comes to dating and relationships in that the individual will get themselves into situations that are dangerous and can end up sleeping around and be at risk of sexually transmitted infections or unplanned pregnancy. Attempts by family members to limit social escapades are usually met with a lot of anger and resistance.

Along with exposing themselves to dangerous situations, the individuals can also present with an inability to assess dangers and consequences of their actions. This can lead to further brain injuries and issues with the police.

All in all, personality changes due to frontal lobe damage present a great challenge to the individual and to those around them. Treatment options are present, though they can be frustratingly limited and getting access to such treatment is a challenge.

Symptoms of Organic Personality Disorder:

- Impulsive poorly thought out behaviour – e.g. purchases, drinking, gambling.
- Disinhibition: being sexually lewd or other inappropriate social behaviour.
- Jocular juvenile behaviour- e.g. pranks, jokes.
- Irritability and sudden loss of temper.
- Poor insight.
- Lacking empathy or consideration for how others feel.
- Changes represent a big change from pre-brain injury behaviour.

MEDICAL MANAGEMENT

On the whole medication has a limited role in the management of behavioural problems as a result of brain injury. Medication on its own cannot eliminate all of the personality problems associated with a frontal lobe injury. However, they can certainly help some issues like agitation and mood in conjunction with psychological and social therapies. Unfortunately, research into this really important area is quite limited in terms of quality, randomised controlled trials. Despite this, a number of medications are widely used in the treatment of aggression and anger as a result of frontal lobe damage.

Antidepressants are often widely used in the treatment of frustration and aggression associated with a brain injury. This is because, as mentioned earlier, in the context of a brain injury, it can be particularly difficult to differentiate depression from other symptoms after brain injury. Personality change, particularly irritability or apathy, is a symptom that is also often seen in depression. As a result, it can be worthwhile giving someone with irritability a trial of an antidepressant to see if this helps with some of the behavioural difficulties. On the whole, the side effects of antidepressant medication are fairly minor and these medications are well tolerated.

Some antiepileptic medications are routinely used as mood stabilisers in bipolar affective disorder. Even though the behaviour seen in bipolar affective disorder is very different to that seen after brain injury, by convention a number of antiepileptic medications have over the years been used with some success for the resulting anger and agitation. Carbamazepine and valproic acid are the most commonly used. Both are well tolerated but require blood tests due to the potential for side effects, particularly in the case of valproic acid which may be associated with development of abnormal liver function tests. Valproate is also associated with congenital birth defects and as such should be avoided in young women who aren't taking contraceptives.

The blood pressure tablet propranolol has also been used for anger problems. Anecdotally, this seems to be of particular benefit in those with explosive and short-lived anger. The drug is also used occasionally in panic disorders and is non-addictive and usually well tolerated. It can cause breathing difficulties in those with asthma and for this reason is usually avoided in people with asthma and those with heart rate abnormalities. The main side effects are lowering of blood pressure, slowing of heart rate and mild drowsiness. Blood pressure is usually monitored and patients prescribed are advised to get up slowly and advise their physician if they feel dizzier when standing or unstable on their feet.

Antipsychotic medications are also used at times in the management of agitation. Many have mood stabilising properties and some, such as quetiapine or olanzapine, also have a sedative effect and can assist with sleep. Some of the older antipsychotics such as haloperidol or newer ones like risperidone, particularly at higher doses, can cause side effects affecting movement such as slowing of walking, tremor, and a sense of restlessness or involuntary movements. These antipsychotics in particular should be avoided being taken in the long-term and families should discuss any concerns about these and other medications with their doctor.

PSYCHOLOGICAL MANAGEMENT

Anger management techniques can also be of benefit in people with irritability after a brain injury. The individuals who benefit from anger management need to have better insight and cognitively need to be able to understand and be open to the rationale of the techniques. There are many types of anger management techniques but the therapist teaching them will start the process through examining the situations that are associated with anger problems. In particular they will be interested in the ABCs: antecedents, behaviour and consequences. Along with the individual, the therapist examines the antecedents or situations that predispose to anger problems. This can be done through the use of diaries or in inpatient facilities through physically observing what factors are associated with loss of temper. The actual behaviours themselves are noted to see if there is a stepwise progression of the behaviour so that caregivers can be on the lookout for signs of impending temper and prevent problems before they develop. Finally, the consequences of behaviour are explored with the individual in order to help them understand and appreciate more fully the effect that their behaviour has both on themselves and others.

CBT can also occasionally be used in individuals with personality changes or behavioural issues after a brain injury. The therapist should be experienced and such therapy would generally need to be individualised and given on a one-to-one basis as there is no 'one size fits all' way for offering CBT.

Supportive psychotherapy or counselling can sometimes be a very helpful psychological treatment for this group of patients. Invariably the behaviours associated with organic personality disorder can lead to a lot of stress and distress for the individual affected. They frequently end up alienating themselves from other individuals and family members. Gentle counselling with an experienced therapist can allow the individual to ventilate how they're feeling. The therapist in a firm and supportive manner also needs to point out the consequences of the individual's impulsive or disinhibited behaviour. Such pointing out of behavioural issues can go a long way towards building or improving some degree of insight.

SOCIAL THERAPIES

Social interventions have the greatest role in the management of personality and behavioural problems due to frontal lobe damage. Fundamentally, those with severe personality and behavioural problems are only as good as the environment in which they live and the supports they have. In daily clinical practice, I usually find that regardless of the severity of brain injury, patients who present with the greatest level of personality and behavioural difficulties are those with the poorest level of supports or who come from chaotic family backgrounds.

The place where the individual is discharged to along with the level of support available is vital in attempting to manage what is often an impossible situation. In cases where a family is unable to or unwilling to manage the brain injury survivor and their behaviour, they may end up having to go into care. The types and levels of supports available vary greatly from place to place and is usually dependent on funding, either from local social services or compensation payouts. At its most basic, the levels of support required can consist of an individual living in their own home with a support worker or home help coming in daily or a number of times per week. In more complex cases the support workers may visit the individual multiple times a day, especially if the taking of medications has to be supervised. Those with more challenging behaviours may need to live somewhere with someone present onsite 24/7, whilst patients with even more challenging behaviours will need to live in a small group home with a carer present 24/7. Individuals with more complex behavioural challenges or medical needs may need to live in care facilities with nursing staff or other professional back-up. Decisions relating to the levels of support and location of supports are invariably quite challenging and are discussed earlier in chapter seven.

PRACTICAL WAYS OF DEALING WITH ORGANIC PERSONALITY DISORDER

General Approaches

- Overstimulation is a major cause of agitation. Overstimulation can be reduced by limiting the amount of noises and music in the home, public and in clinical settings. For example, rather than having meals in public areas, it's best to have them in quieter places where the distraction is less. Similarly, too many visitors can be physically and cognitively taxing.

- Imposing firm rules and boundaries. The individuals who have worse outcomes after a brain injury are those who come from chaotic households in the first place. The individual should be given clear rules on returning home. Pre-brain injury activities such as going out socialising late, taking drugs or drinking alcohol should be avoided and it's important to regularly remind the individual/s affected about these ground rules.

Anger and Agitation

- Avoid walking on egg shells or over-indulging. It is easy for family members to be so relieved that a loved one has survived a devastating brain injury that they give them free rein and tolerate and minimise behavioural problems. Ultimately this strategy tends to encourage further behavioural problems and isn't fruitful.

- Being aware of the causes of agitation and aggression is important. It is useful to note what factors are associated with the individual losing their temper so they can be avoided. Do they become angrier when overstimulated, when they are being asked difficult questions, or when others aren't listening to them or talk down to them and treat them like a child?

- Agitation and anger can frequently be associated with some of the following factors. Is there any evidence that these factors play an important role in development of anger?
- Fatigue: is the individual overly tired? At every point in the recovery journey fatigue can be problematic. Even relatively simple tasks like going to new places or trips by car can be fatigue provoking.
- Are they hungry or thirsty?
- Are they bored and being made to do something that they don't want to be doing?
- Do they feel threatened or demeaned by others in some way – is their anger a rational response to a real or perceived slight?
- Are they scared? Life with a brain injury can be scary, especially if there are challenges with short-term memory or speech or communication problems where expressing that fear is not possible.

Impulsive Behaviours

- If the individual has friends that were a bad influence pre-injury, it is worthwhile trying to limit access to these individuals or supervising their visits.
- Substance misuse through drugs or alcohol is a disaster in acquired brain injury. Family and friends need to deliberately limit access to drink or drugs. In cases where there is evidence of addiction present, the individual needs to be referred to local addiction services.
- Social media and the internet can be great for individuals after a brain injury in terms of allowing them to communicate with friends or relatives. However, it may be wise for the family to be cognisant about the less savoury aspects of social media and in particular access to situations where the individual may be used or abused or have access to unsavoury websites. The family should therefore be mindful of such risks and if they are concerned about the individual being exposed to risks or being

abused or harassed they should liaise with the individual and consider imposing limits or safeguards in terms of internet access.

- Access to money: if the individual is prone to overspending and purchasing drugs or alcohol, the family need to discuss with social workers or the medical team whether access to funds can be restricted, particularly if there is evidence that the individual is vulnerable and lacks capacity in their purchases.

Disinhibition in Social Situations

- If there is evidence that the individual is more disinhibited in certain busy social situations, for example in church services, cinemas, or busy shopping centres, it's worthwhile avoiding such settings or limiting them to times when they are less crowded.
- If there are particular people that the individual is more likely to be disinhibited with, for example the obese, children, members of ethnic minorities etc, it might be worthwhile attempting to limit the public situations where the individual is exposed to such groups.

Loss of Empathy

- Self-protection: caring for an individual with personality change due to brain injury is highly exhausting and stressful. Burnout can develop in a slow and insidious way. Be aware that you are not an inexhaustible resource and take care of yourself both physically and emotionally. It is not without its joys, however.

If in doubt get advice from the brain injury team or from others who have looked after those with a brain injury or from Headway or other brain injury support groups.

CASE HISTORY: THE CHILDISH FATHER

Michael was a responsible 34-year-old married father of three children and a builder until his brain injury, when his car careered off the road on his way to work early one icy morning. In addition to a number of fractures of his ribs and other bones, he sustained a severe head injury. He was unconscious for a number of weeks and was transferred to his local neuroscience centre for treatment as he had a large clot and severe bruising around his frontal lobes.

After the acute phase of his treatment was completed, he was transferred to a rehabilitation unit. He spent a number of weeks there and, whilst his family noted that he appeared a bit different, they did not have any concerns due to the fact that he was in a hospital environment and he had been through so much.

It was not until he was discharged home that it became apparent to his family the extent of how his personality had changed. Prior to his injury, Michael was a good-humoured and jovial character, but he was an extremely responsible husband, parent and worker. He was a devoted husband to his wife, Jacquie, of over ten years. He was a kind father to his three children, the youngest of whom was just 5 years old.

When he returned home, Jacquie felt that he was somewhat ex-citable, a little bit like their younger son, when in a new environment. Jacquie, however, put this down to the fact that Michael had been in rehabilitation for so long that he was just simply glad to be at home. She noticed that he had a tendency to monopolise the conversation at the dinner table and to just talk about himself all of the time. He ap-peared to be less interested in the children and was insensitive to how Jacquie herself was coping. She also noticed that when he would play with the children, he used to try and beat them and win at games. The older children in particular found his behaviour difficult to deal with, and increasingly used to try and avoid spending time with him. Jacquie also noted that Michael had tantrums if things were not done quickly enough for him. Due to the fact that his sense of smell was poor as a result of the accident, his appetite could be variable. Generally, he had a preference for sweet things, and he also used to steal some of the crisps and sweets that she had bought for their children. When she tried to discuss his behaviour with him, he would become irritable or simply laugh at her. Whilst he always was a jovial man, she increasingly noticed that he had a tendency to laugh everything off, and to also repeat jokes which were not in any way funny, over and over again at the dinner table, and in other social outlets. He also tended to swear and use rude words in front of the children. Things came to a head and she finally sought help when she was awoken one morning at 6:00 a.m. to see her husband out in the back garden kicking a football wearing pyjamas. She realised that he had changed from being a responsible husband and father, to being more childish than their children.

What happened to Michael is typical of organic personality disorder. An often-observed situation in cases such as this is that pre-brain injury personality traits become magnified and exaggerated after the injury and the individual becomes a parody of themselves. In the case of Michael, pre-brain injury he was a jovial character. After, he became overly jocular and made lots of irreverent and often inappropriate jokes.

Management of someone like Michael is difficult and mainly involves offering lots of support to his wife and kids. Medication has a limited role in this kind of case and the most important input is in the form of social and psychological supports both for Michael and his family. Michael would benefit from regular input from a support worker to try and give him a schedule that involves him getting out of the family home and being as active as possible. In the case of someone like Michael, his behaviour is worse when he is bored or left to his own devices. It is therefore important to keep him safely and reasonably occupied whilst at the same time ensuring that he is not over-stimulated and therefore fatigued.

Help for the family as a whole is particularly important in cases such as this. Headway, the brain charity, have some very good booklets that explain brain injury to children. In addition, counselling for the children and especially the partner/spouse can be very useful.

CASE HISTORY: THE ANGRY YOUNG MAN

Paul is a 19-year-old young man who had a very chaotic upbringing. His father was an alcoholic and his mother, whilst she did her best, was incapable of imposing rules and boundaries on his bad behaviour. As a result, since his early teenage years, he was in trouble with school authorities and was suspended and expelled from a number of schools. He got into trouble with the police for antisocial behaviour, drug and alcohol use, and aggression towards others.

Paul sustained his brain injury as a result of being beaten up by two large men. Whilst the assailants were never caught, it was felt by many that they had beaten Paul up severely after he had failed to pay them money for drugs that he had consumed.

Paul sustained a very severe brain injury and was unconscious for over a week. He had multiple bleeds in his brain and had to have part of his skull removed due to swelling. He was confused, agitated and aggressive for a long time after regaining consciousness.

After his physical symptoms were treated, he was transferred to a rehabilitation unit, though throughout his time in the unit he showed evidence of severe behavioural challenges. He frequently would get annoyed with staff or other patients if he felt that they had insulted or upset him in any way. His temper was explosive and quick, although he had little in the way of regret after he upset or hurt someone. He was discharged to the family home with a care package in place. However, his parents soon found that they were unable to control his behaviour. As he became physically stronger and better from his other physical injuries, he started going out. He would leave the house at all hours. Sometimes he would end up going drinking. Sometimes he would meet up with former friends and sometimes he would just simply wander aimlessly. The relationship with his former girlfriend, who had stuck by him throughout his inpatient stay, broke down after he made threats against her, and attempted to sexually assault her. His mother admitted that he was constantly shouting and screaming at her, slamming doors and stamping his feet. He occasionally threatened to hit his father, with whom he had always had a tense relationship. Social services became increasingly concerned about his behaviour. He was placing himself in significant danger and seemed unaware of the consequences of his actions. He ended up being assaulted a further time, again due to some of his antisocial behaviour. In the end, it was felt necessary to section him under the Mental Health Act and commit him to a local psychiatric unit for assessment purposes.

Managing someone like Paul is especially difficult. Risks in such cases are substantial and individuals can get themselves into all kinds of difficulties with the police, local criminals, neighbours, relatives and friends. Their lives can very easily spiral out of control and without any support or patience from family or social services they can seriously endanger the safety of themselves and others. It is important to note that in cases like Paul's, his pre-injury behaviour was far from ideal and he was far from ever being a model citizen. Indeed, his brain injury was probably as a result of his chaotic lifestyle. In his case, his pre-injury wild side was exaggerated and due to his young age, his frontal lobes were still immature meaning he was automatically at a disadvantage.

Longer-term management of individuals like Paul consists of integrated care between social, mental health and potentially police services. Individuals like Paul are only as good as the placement and the supports that they receive. Serious consideration would need to be made for him being discharged from section to a supported living or care home facility.

CASE HISTORY: APATHY

Mary was a sprightly and energetic 63-year-old grandmother. She was well known for always being on the go, and it was a family joke that she could never be found at home due to the fact that she was always out, either at the Women's Institute, volunteering, or at various fitness classes. Unfortunately, whilst out shopping one day, she suffered a cardiac arrest. She was collapsed on the ground for a number of minutes before a passer-by, who was trained in CPR, started giving her chest compressions. She was transferred to a local hospital and her family were delighted and relieved to hear that she survived.

However, as she began her recovery they noticed that she had a very poor short-term memory and would not remember who had been in to see her. They also noted that, whereas in the past she was very interested in what was going on with her grandchildren, she seemed far more disinterested. The severity of her symptoms was especially noticeable when she was discharged home. She needed considerable encouragement in her daily activities and would sit in the same place in the living room all day, and not move. She was very disinterested when she was taken to group settings, whereas in the past she used to enjoy herself. Overall, her family felt that she was a completely different person and a shell of her former self.

Cases like Mary's are particularly distressing for family members. Families frequently may wonder if their loved ones, in situations such as this, are depressed. Antidepressant medications may indeed often be prescribed though to limited benefit. Other medications such as stimulants are also occasionally used, though again results can be limited. Psychological interventions are similarly fruitless and there are limited interventions available other than that of supporting the family in coming to terms with their very different loved one. Apathy syndromes are reflective of widespread brain damage and can be a feature of damage as a result of a cardiac arrest or when vast areas of the frontal lobes are damaged.

CHAPTER FOURTEEN

Post-concussion Syndrome

POST-CONCUSSION SYMPTOMS

Head injuries vary considerably in severity. As already described in chapter four, the severity is graded by duration of how long one is 'knocked out' after a head injury, the level of consciousness as defined by the Glasgow Coma Scale (GCS), the duration of confusion after regaining consciousness and the duration of Post-traumatic Amnesia (PTA). Mild, moderate and severe brain injuries can therefore be quite well defined based on these criteria.

However, even after so-called mild brain injuries, debilitating symptoms can be experienced. This is hardly surprising since even these patients can have subtle abnormalities on brain scans and the brain itself may not function at the same level in the immediate aftermath. Brain scans used in ordinary clinical practice tend to show how a brain looks rather than how it works. Just because there is no evidence on a scan of obvious abnormalities doesn't necessarily mean that the brain is working at prime condition. The real purpose of a brain scan is to show is that there is no evidence of problems that require urgent medical intervention.

After any brain injury, there can be subtle changes to attention or concentration, or other physical or emotional symptoms. These diverse symptoms are generally referred to as post-concussion symptoms.

A physical symptom commonly seen after a brain injury is headache. The headache can vary in severity and can sometimes be related to taking too many painkillers – called analgesic overuse headache.

Dizziness is also a common feature after a head injury and can be associated with tinnitus – hearing a buzzing in one's ears. The individuals affected may also complain of loud noises or bright lights hurting them and as a result they may shy away from chaotic environments. Fatigue is a very important symptom and this isn't helped by the fact that the sleep pattern can also be strongly impaired. The fatigue may be present all the time meaning the individual will find that even little chores or tasks are enough to overwhelm them. Being overly tired can also worsen emotional instability and lead to irritability and upset.

Cognitively, the individual may complain of poor attention and concentration. As a result, they will report forgetfulness and may misplace objects. The most common complaint relating to cognition is that of feeling 'muzzy' or less sharp about things. As a result, they can be more forgetful and have a tendency to make silly mistakes, for example looking for a mobile phone only to discover that it is in their hand or placing food items into an oven when it was the fridge that it was meant to be placed. They may inadvertently misplace objects or find that they have left lights on, doors open or water running. The individual frequently in such cases thinks that they are going mad or developing a dementia or other serious memory problem. Of course, these are things we can all do from time to time, particularly if we're stressed or tired and it's important to be mindful of that fact and to not be too hard on ourselves, especially in the early aftermath after and head injury. Those individuals whose work requires a high degree of concentration (teachers, managers, businesspeople, air traffic controllers etc.) will be more aware of these differences than those who work in less cognitively demanding jobs.

From a behavioural perspective, individuals affected will report irritability and may have problems with losing their temper, especially if fatigued or overstimulated. They can also be more emotional and become tearful with little provocation and may complain of feeling down and low in mood.

Psychologically, the individual may feel useless and become concerned that their personality is irrevocably changed forever. They will frequently say 'I'm not the same person' and feel that they have changed totally.

Post-concussion Symptoms

- headaches
- dizziness
- fatigue
- tinnitus
- blurred vision
- fatigue
- noise sensitivity
- light sensitivity
- irritability
- anxiety
- insomnia
- low mood
- feeling emotional
- poor concentration
- forgetfulness
- apathy

OUTCOME

The good news about post-concussion symptoms is that they generally resolve in most people after a period of around six months. However, a substantial minority can experience ongoing symptoms for a far longer period after what frequently at first appears to have been a trivial injury. The symptoms in this group are usually more anxiety and mood associated than the purely physical symptoms that are observed in the early aftermath. Some studies have shown an association with other psychosomatic disorders like chronic pain, fibromyalgia, and irritable bowel syndrome. There is also an association with previous depressive and anxiety disorders.

TREATMENT

The best treatment of post-concussion symptoms is to treat the individual symptoms and allow time to enact the cure and give lots of reassurance. Virtually everyone after a brain injury will have some degree of fatigue and poor concentration and it is important to allow time for the brain to heal. The affected individual should take care not to try and get back to work too soon and should heed their body and rest if they feel tired and fatigued rather than fighting the tiredness with consequent knock-on effects on irritability, mood and confidence. Individual symptoms like low mood, anxiety, headaches and sleep problems can be treated by general practitioners and easily respond to treatment with medications such as painkillers and/or antidepressants. Those with more severe and chronic symptoms may require more specialised help from neuropsychiatry or benefit from a referral for counselling.

Advice for Family Members on Dealing with Post-concussion Syndrome Problems:

- Normalise symptoms but don't over dramatize: any knock to the head will have some short-terms symptoms. Therefore, it's important to reassure the family member affected of the constellation of physical, cognitive and emotional symptoms and not point out their failings.
- Don't get preoccupied with deadlines to be better or deadlines to be back at work – people take very different amounts of time to get better.
- Look up books and articles on post-concussion syndrome and be aware of the various symptoms present and reassure the individual that they're not going mad, their symptoms are not unusual and the role that rest and time have in recovery. Avoid internet forums devoted to post-concussion syndrome however, as these often present worst-case scenarios and don't serve to help one's confidence.

- Be aware that some medications, like amitriptyline, which can be given for pain, may be associated with reversible cognitive side effects. And be mindful of the s risks of taking too much paracetamol or other painkillers.
- Support individuals in taking lots of naps and rests if fatigue is an issue at the start.

CASE HISTORY: POST-CONCUSSION SYNDROME

Georgina is a 48-year-old woman who, in her mid-40s, discovered cycling. She had a trusted mountain bike and was always out cycling on country roads and mountain paths during the weekends. She was quite a responsible individual, and always wore a helmet. However, one day, whilst cycling down a path, her bike hit a pothole and she was thrown from it. She was cycling with others on that day, and her companions noted that she had a momentary loss of consciousness. When she came to, she was dazed for a couple of seconds, but was otherwise not confused.

She was seen at her local casualty department and was discharged the same day. However, after the incident, she felt that she was not herself. She complained of ringing in her ears and headaches. She also felt that her balance was affected and she felt less confident. In addition, she complained of severe fatigue and stopped exercising. She felt that her memory was poor and found it harder to concentrate. She also complained of low mood.

Over a number of months, her physical symptoms of headaches and dizziness improved, but she continued to complain of memory problems and fatigue. Four months later she remained quite debilitated. She felt that she was no longer her same self. She believed that she had changed as a person. She was so concerned about her symptoms that she went to her GP and was referred to a neurologist. However, a subsequent brain scan showed no evidence of any changes.

Mild head injuries like Georgina's can frequently be anything but mild. The physical symptoms of the post-concussional state can be alarming, and reassurance from professionals that the injury was trivial can seem condescending. The physical symptoms frequently dissipate after a number of months but residual cognitive symptoms can remain for some time.

CHAPTER FIFTEEN

Stages in Response to Trauma: Coping as a family

COPING WITH THE LOSS

Irish folktales frequently refer to the idea of the 'changeling', where a healthy child was spirited away by the fairies and in its place was left an identical looking but different and unhealthy replacement.[14] The family knew that their loved one was not present but were powerless to effect any change to the situation. So they looked after their new unwell youngster whilst mourning all the time for their child and those better days of the past.

ABI can present a similar scenario for families. Not all mourning is for the dead. Not all loss is felt by the bereaved. And in all our lives we suffer the pangs of grief as the price of being alive, of loving, and if we're lucky, being loved. When we mourn, we yearn not just for the loved one but for the order of those seemingly distant happier days, we miss our naïve hope for the future, we miss the way we felt, and indeed we miss the loss of ourselves in being part of an "other half". In an instant, the world has changed, and we must struggle to find a new direction and new path for ourselves and our families.

---

[14] The interested reader might enjoy the poem *The Stolen Child* by W.B. Yeats which eloquently describes the folklore surrounding the idea from the point of view of the child.

Many professionals and books refer to the Kubler-Ross model of grief. A Swiss–American psychiatrist, Elizabeth Kubler-Ross, developed a five stages of grief model to describe a survivor's means of dealing with the death of a loved one.

Denial: A belief that the ABI is minor and that new disabilities aren't present

Anger: Annoyance and anger towards the loved one, the circumstances of the trauma, and those involved in the care of the loved one.

Bargaining: A belief that through certain actions the ABI can be magically undone.

Depression: A loss of all hope. Being struck down by the enormity of the situation.

Acceptance: A gradual embracing of the new normal situation post brain injury.

Whilst originally described in the context of bereavement, it has also been used to put into words the means of coping with a number of other situations and losses in life. Her ideas have become part of mainstream culture – being mentioned even in a classic episode of the Simpsons. However, like any model, it is far from perfect and given that loss is not a one size fits all phenomenon, it is blind to the special circumstances of the trauma of ABI.

A special feature of coping with a family member surviving a brain injury is its incompleteness and lack of closure. There is no death; there is life but it is an unfamiliar one. A form that is at once similar but not quite the same. In milder forms of ABI, a family may face a loved one who just requires some additional supports and assistance. In more severe forms of ABI, physical disability may involve the toil of readjusting one's house to cope with wheelchairs, hoists, and the invasions of an army of carers coming in and out. Organic personality disorder in particular is traumatic in that the loved one is at once physically similar but so different in their personality, their lack of insight, and irresponsibility. The loss of empathy in particular and the changes in the dynamics of the relationship from being a spouse, parent, sibling, child to feeling that one is now a referee and supervisor is particularly difficult. The feelings of resentment and frustration, all the while, having to be supressed. Whilst, at the same time suffering the platitudes of being told by others that one is lucky that the loved one is still alive – and at once feeling invalidated in one's feelings of grief and exhaustion.

Traumas are invariably sudden, unannounced, unexpected and overwhelming. For most, the occurrence of an ABI is similar. Notwithstanding the feelings of loss associated with a brain injury, a more appropriate way of viewing an ABI is from the viewpoint of a severe psychological trauma for a family.

Psychological trauma is experienced and relived in five different but complementary (and rhyming) ways: freeze, flight, fight, fright or please. At different stages of the journey, different feelings may predominate. Personality or circumstances of the trauma may mean that some are more likely to experience one form of these than others. Unlike the Kubler-Ross stages, there is no neat progression towards a form of resolution. Healing is best described by the words of the late Rose Kennedy: "It has been said, time heals all wounds. I do not agree. The wounds remain. In time, the mind, protecting its sanity, covers them with scar tissue and the pain lessens. But it is never gone."

Freeze

An overbearing sense of shock is often the first response to news that a loved one has been in an accident or suffered an injury. This can physically manifest in a gut-wrenching sensation or feeling faint. Psychologically, things feel unreal, like a dream in which one is watching an unfamiliar scene and is powerless to do anything. Emotionally, the individual feels detached and time seems to stop. The memory of the whole scene is burned into the brain but in a different manner to that in which normal memories form. The scene is recalled in a disjointed fashion with a jumble of images, feelings and sounds that is out of kilter with the actual sequence of events. Important information on what actually happened may be lost or repressed.

Afterwards, the individual may feel unsure of the exact details but can find that reminders of what happened can provoke sudden and sometimes incapacitating reactions. The reminders vary greatly and can be sights, smells, sounds or scenarios similar to the trauma-invoking event. The individual may be aware of the link between the trigger and the past trauma but often is unaware and unsure of what is provoking reactions. The reactions themselves take the form of various symptoms of anxiety including racing heart, shortness of breath, tremulousness, tiredness, fear or sensations of derealisation. Derealisation can be very subtle and involve the individual 'zoning one' or appearing to go into their own world.

Flight

The response of some to bad news is 'flight' or running away. Avoidance and denial can be lifetime responses by many. Denial is a psychological defence mechanism whereby the individual pretends to themselves that nothing is wrong and that nothing has happened. They can carry on regardless of what happened and present with an incongruent and inappropriate manner that is grossly out of keeping with the circumstances they are in. In the context of the ABI of a loved one this can take the form of a family member physically running away and avoiding hospital visits.

Toxic hope or toxic positivity represent other flights of fantasy that may be observed. At a certain level, hope is essential after a brain injury. Outcomes are uncertain and even experienced professionals can be unable to answer the important questions in relation to the future. Hope can also be a motivating factor in the long dark night of rehabilitation. It's easy to fear that when hope dies, any prospect for improvement also dies. However, when that level of ambition is at odds with the practical reality, then the ultimate victim is the person with the ABI who feels that their failure to achieve is ultimately down to them. Such hope can also set up rehabilitation services to fail – any gains are discounted and lost in the pile of expectations. Meetings with professionals can rapidly feel like a battle of wills and one in which the treating team seems to consistently downplay the family's aspiration.

Whilst not agreeing with Nietzsche, in the case of toxic hope, he had a point when he said that it "is the worst of all evils, because it prolongs man's torments".

Fight

Fight or projecting one's annoyance onto another is a very human way of dealing with trauma. Anger as a reaction towards a brain injury is more than reasonable – particularly if the brain injury occurred directly as a result of the action or inaction of another individual. Family members can feel a variety of contradictory feelings of sadness, guilt, resentment and love towards their loved one, particularly if the same loved one was in some way partly responsible for their own brain injury. This is often the case if the loved one was an alcoholic, drug user or had an impulsive personality which directly led to the brain injury. A sense of frustration at their role in causing their brain injury and the inability to express that upset directly can lead to others getting the brunt of the anger in the crossfire.

It is easy and trite to point out the shortcomings of chronic rage and in particular the likelihood of displacing that vexation to other thoroughly innocent individuals. In daily medical practice, I continue to find amazing the degree of hostility that some family members occasionally can display towards staff. Nursing staff or poorly paid support staff are often at the receiving end of behaviour from upset and furious family members that would not be acceptable in other areas of life. Whilst most therapists, clinicians and nurses are professional enough to see that the irritation of the relatives is displaced anger, such feelings are by its nature toxic to the collaborative relationship that is essential between treating and rehab teams and the family to get the best possible outcome. Petulant outbursts do nothing to improve or facilitate that relationship and no professional is completely immune to the constant and hostile onslaught of bullying from a family. I have seen staff reduced to tears by such family members and have observed a collective groan from staff when such family members enter the ward or rehabilitation unit. The current status of complaints procedures and tolerance of irrational and unreasonable demands means that complaints receive a degree of attention that they frequently ill deserve. Such complaints, as well as slowly sapping staff's motivation, contribute to burnout and are a desperate waste of resources in national health and social services that are already squeezed financially. Family members who themselves feel such anger can do well to address it by seeking their own psychological supports.

Fright

Anxiety can be a particular problem in relatives after a family member has a brain injury. Worrying is normal. However, for some it can be both excessive and detrimental. The constellation of incomplete information on prognosis, variability on a daily basis and physical exhaustion is an incubator for developing anxiety in the most calm of individuals. As described in greater detail in chapter twelve, anxiety can take many forms. Awareness and early support are important and can be lifesaving.

Please

Psychological tests on laboratory animals found that after prolonged trauma and punishments, the animals become stuck and stopped trying to avoid trauma. In a similar way, people after constant stressors can stop fighting back and become apathetic and resigned to their situation. Patients with chronic mental illness in particular can lose their sense of self and become passive to the demands of others and ignore their own needs. This can also happen to family members after any form of trauma, including ABI. Clinically, such individuals are great to work with. They agree with everything the professionals request. They diligently care for their loved one. They don't request additional supports. As individuals, they disappear and exist solely to please others. In the end, they become so estranged from their own feelings that they develop other mental health or addiction problems or they burn out and develop physical illness. In a world where balance is key, the need to please needs to be balanced with a consciousness of one's own needs.

Mental Health and Well-being of Relatives/Carers

Brain injury is traumatic for the whole family. One study of the mental health of relatives found that 73% had symptoms of depression and 55% had symptoms of anxiety after the injury. Rates of depression remain high for many years after the injury and may be compounded by development of alcohol or other substance misuse problems.

The amount of care given informally by relatives has been estimated in the UK to be worth £119 billion annually in 2011. A 2012 survey by the brain injury charity Headway found devastating psychological, physical and social consequences for carers. More than half of the carers were either retired or unemployed as a result of their carer duties. Over 70% had suffered financial loss and less than a quarter received any carer allowances. Only 7% had a social worker and most felt that they didn't receive sufficient support. Over 50% of carers were providing more than 40 hours of care per week and most felt socially isolated and had lost friends as a result of their carer role.

The same survey found that less than a third had received a carer's assessment and half were quite unaware they had a right to get such an assessment.

Carer's Assessment

The rights of carers of individuals with a disability to receive a formal assessment from the local authority is enshrined in the Care Act 2014 in England and other similar legislation in Scotland, Wales and Northern Ireland. Any individual with a carer role has the right to such an assessment which aims to determine whether the carer is entitled to any help or assistance from the State. The assessment consists of a professional from the local authority looking at the amount of care an individual is providing and the impact on their own life. If deemed eligible, the council may offer additional support which may take a variety of forms including day care centre, support worker input, or respite care, to name but a few. The local authority may also complete a financial assessment to see whether an additional contribution is required to implement the new plan.

Signs of Carer Burnout

Caregiver burnout is the name given to a state of physical and emotional exhaustion as a result of feeling chronically overwhelmed by carer duties. Carer burnout affects the carer but also other family members and the individual who is being cared for. Symptoms of burnout develop insidiously and can be physical and emotional, or a creeping resentment towards the person being cared for.

The signs are many but include:

- Physical symptoms of stress or depression – insomnia, reduced appetite, weight loss, feeling tired all the time, listlessness, poor concentration.
- Emotional symptoms such as tearfulness, irritability, panic, anxiety, feelings of resentment or low mood.
- Excessive use of alcohol or prescription medications such as diazepam or sleeping tablets.
- Feeling out of control.
- Becoming neglectful of the person being cared for or shouting at them or being physically rough with them.

The most important thing to do if you are feeling overburdened is to seek help and tell someone, be it a family member, friend or professional such as a GP or Social Worker. Untreated, carer burnout can progress to serious mental and physical problems; and early recognition, and treatment and support is vital.

General Advice for Family Members

- Be aware that the whole process of recovering after a brain injury and rehabilitation is a marathon and not a sprint. Some days will be good and many days will be bad. A lot of the time there will be the sense of one step forward and two steps back.

- Be aware that the needs of other family members, especially children doesn't disappear after a loved one gets a brain injury.

- Be open and honest with children about the nature of brain injury of their family members. Headway produces a very good booklet for children explaining brain injury.

- Own your feelings. Feelings of resentment are the mind's way of indicating that you're feeling over-whelmed and trapped. If you are developing significant emotional responses make note of them and ponder why you are feeling that way and figure out what you can do to deal with those feelings.

- Be aware that you can feel anger and annoyance to-wards the loved one who sustained the brain injury and their role in getting a brain injury in the first place. Try not to take such feelings out on them but don't be shy about being honest if the loved one, for example, starts drinking alcohol or engaging in other impulsive acts again.

- Do look after your own health and well-being and be open to taking days off visiting – going into a hospital daily can be desperately draining and the feelings of exhaustion build up slowly and often unnoticed.

- Try and meet and get support from other individuals or families who are in a similar position. Local or online support groups can be very helpful in this regard. It's difficult to beat the informal support obtained by making friends with other families who have a loved one in the same rehabilitation unit.

- Don't be a hero – seek help before your role as a carer becomes overwhelming, particularly if there aren't other family members available to lighten the load

CHAPTER SIXTEEN

Frequently Asked Questions

Am I at high risk of brain damage if I get a further tap to my head?

One of the great misconceptions after the brain injury, or if someone suffers a skull fracture, is that their brain is now suddenly like an egg shell so that even minor taps to the head can cause brain damage. The worst thing that can be done to an individual after suffering a brain injury, is that they are wrapped in cotton wool.

It's been a while since my brain injury, yet I'm getting worse. Could this be the brain injury?

It is very common for an individual, either after leaving hospital, or as they become more and more independent, to feel more fatigued or more forgetful. This is because the controlled environment in hospital or in the rehabilitation unit is artificial and not as cognitively or physically demanding as home. The initial period of being discharged home is associated with a honeymoon period. Many can feel like they are almost back to normal initially. It is not until they gradually start to try more and more, that they encounter problems such as fatigue, irritability and notice the depth of their concentration and memory problems. There are many reasons for someone feeling that they are getting more forgetful after a brain injury, including depression and low mood problems The most frequent cause I find, however, is that the individuals are expecting far too much of themselves at far too early a stage.

My neurosurgeon said that I would be as good as I would get after a year, and that after that, I would not improve. Is that true?

The one- or two-year rule is something that is frequently said to patients after a brain injury by varying medical specialists. Given that every single brain injury is completely different, and that people's circumstance and known physical health and well-being are very different, it is very difficult to have a hard rule of thumb as to when it is possible to say that an individual is 'as good as they will be' after a brain injury. The most noticeable period of gains and improvement will occur within the first couple of months to the first 12 months. That said, individuals continue to improve, albeit at a lower rate afterwards. People can continue to make ongoing steady and/or slow improvements after a brain injury for many, many years.

When can I drive again?

Anyone with a driving licence in the UK is legally required to notify the Driver and Vehicle Licensing Agency (DVLA) following a brain injury. If they fail to do this their insurance is invalid. An individual is not able to drive until after they have received approval from the DVLA. The DVLA may ask your doctor to complete a questionnaire. Sometimes they may also request a formal driving assessment. **Driving a vehicle without having obtained prior permission from the DVLA is against the law and can result in either a fine or imprisonment.**

Driving itself is a very cognitively and physically demanding exercise requiring high levels of attention and concentration, as well as requiring good problem-solving and visual and auditory skills. Some of the medications given in the aftermath of a brain injury can significantly affect attention and concentration and can lead to sedation. Individuals who develop epilepsy after a brain injury have an additional barrier to returning to driving again.

If the DVLA states that you have permission to drive again, ideally you should start on a very graded and phased basis, preferably with a family member or friend present. For those whose confidence is affected, it can be worthwhile arranging to have some additional driving lessons. The local branch of Headway often has a list of drivers that are particularly skilled in training individuals with brain injuries. You should initially drive around local areas for short periods at non-peak times. This is to improve your driving skills but also to improve your overall confidence.

When can I fly?

There are no hard and fast rules as to when someone will be able to fly but if in doubt ask your consultant or doctor. It is up to your consultant and also your airline as to when you are considered fit to fly. If you have had surgery, it is best to wait at least six weeks. If the individual suffers from significant behavioural or other challenges after the brain injury, including epilepsy, it is advisable for the family to inform the airline. Similarly, if getting travel insurance, it is best to declare the brain injury, or else the insurance may be invalid. Metal detectors at the airport should not affect any coils or clips.

When can I go out alone?

Again, there are no hard and fast rules as to when individuals should be able to go out alone. Ideally, people with more severe memory problems or behavioural problems should go out accompanied by family members or other professionals in the immediate aftermath of their injuries. With time, they can increasingly venture out unaccompanied around local areas. It is recommended to seek the advice from an occupational therapist as to road safety and, in particular, in terms of crossing roads. Similarly, the individual should have a mobile phone on them at all times if they are going out.

When can I play sport?

As well as being a social activity that is good for the cardiovascular system, and for overall health and mental well-being, sport almost certainly has benefits for cognition as well. Following the aftermath of a brain injury, however, it is important to initially only play sport at a very gentle intensity and to gradually build up. Fatigue is a problem after brain injury and being bedbound in hospital for prolonged periods of time naturally leads to a reduction in muscle bulk. This means that risks of injuries are higher, particularly if someone engages in strenuous exercise too soon. Weightlifting or significant gym exercise can raise intracranial pressure and need to be avoided. Similarly, strenuous long-distance running and cycling should also be avoided initially.

Team contact sports such as soccer, where the individual heads a ball, or rugby, or hockey, should also be avoided. Any return to such sports should be discussed with your physiotherapist or doctor.

When can I start having sex again?

Normal sexual activity can be resumed once the individual feels up to it. However, they should be aware that some of the medications that are given after a brain injury, particularly painkillers or antidepressants, can sometimes affect sexual performance. Similarly, damage to the pituitary gland can affect hormone levels and cause reduced sex drive.

When can I commence drinking alcohol again?

After a brain injury, the brain is particularly sensitive to the effects of alcohol. Even small amounts can be enough to make an individual very intoxicated. Alcohol can also interact with some of the medications commonly given, particularly painkillers. In addition, drinking alcohol – particularly at higher quantities – increases the risks of further brain injuries through falls, assaults or further accidents. It is therefore best to avoid alcohol for as long as possible after a brain injury. Any subsequent drinking should be moderate, and binge-drinking really should be avoided.

When can I return to work?

The timing of return to work depends greatly upon the severity of the brain injury. One of the greatest challenges of brain injuries is that frequently people wish to return to work too soon, and this leads to an unsuccessful return, which dents the individual's confidence, and delays a successful return to work. Any return to work after a brain injury needs to be in consultation with your company's occupational health department, and your own consultant or general practitioner. A return to work needs to be on a graded basis, with the individual doing a couple of hours a couple of times a week initially, before gradually increasing. Even the simple day-to-day tasks of getting to work and interacting with one's colleagues can be sufficiently exhausting, particularly in those who already have fatigue problems after a brain injury.

Can I take illicit/recreational drugs?
Recreational drug use is a very bad idea for individuals who have suffered a brain injury. Drugs such as cocaine affect the blood pressure within the brain and can also cause strokes. Similarly, drugs such as amphetamines and MDMA affect blood pressure. Cannabis use may also have a role in development of psychotic symptoms.

When can I return to school or education?
Similar to a return to work, a return to education needs to be done in conjunction with teachers, lecturers or educational supervisors. In some cases, additional support may be required in the form of a notetaker, extra time at exams, or further supports. Any return to education needs, again, to be done on a graded basis.

How do I get advice on benefits?
The best way of getting advice on benefits and other entitlements after a brain injury is to liaise with a Citizens Advice Bureau, or to speak with a social worker if your rehabilitation team has one. The process of completing forms for benefits and obtaining other support is a minefield that is challenging at the best of times. If you do not have access to a social worker or a Citizens Advice Bureau, it is a good idea to liaise with your local head injury or other brain injury voluntary group, and obtain some advocacy advice from them.

How do I meet other individuals with brain injuries and obtain further information and advice?
There are numerous organisations, both national and local, in the United Kingdom and in other countries that provide excellent support for individuals after having suffered a brain injury. Headway is proba-

bly the best known of these, although at a local level many other organisations exist. Your treating rehabilitation team should have some
knowledge about such organisations, and they should be able to sign-
post you to them. Failing that, it is always worthwhile looking up local
support groups and organisations online. Such organisations have a
buddy system whereby it is possible to meet and discuss the challenges
of life after a brain injury with another brain injury survivor. Some
hospitals and rehabilitation units have established volunteer programmes to provide support and advice for other inpatients with brain
injuries.

What are the best ways of ensuring best recovery after a brain injury?

Individuals and family members commonly ask this question. Obviously, there are no hard and fast answers to it. Many individuals frequently use crossword puzzles and puzzle books to try and improve
brain function. Whilst the actual scientific benefits of this are ques-
tionable, certainly there is truth in the old adage 'use it or lose it'. Use
of puzzles, jigsaws and reading can all be of benefit, particularly if the
individual enjoys doing this. A healthy diet with some exercise and
good fatigue management are also essential. In clinical practice, I have
always found that one of the best means of improving recovery is to
avoid some of the habits that may have been a contributory factor to
the development of a brain injury in the first place, particularly if alcoholism has been a challenge. In virtually all cases of brain injury,
avoidance or certainly minimisation of alcohol is essential. Promotion
of good mental health and psychological well-being is also helpful in
improving overall prognosis.

CHAPTER SEVENTEEN

Winning the War: Practical Solutions to Maximising Recovery Potential

Since no brain injury is exactly the same, advice for maximising progress after a brain injury varies greatly from person to person. Some of the advice in this chapter is based on sound scientific evidence. Much of it, however, is based on a mixture of common sense, experience and clinical judgement. Some of the advice will be more practicable and realistic for some severities of ABI than others. Readers and their family members are therefore advised to pick and choose from the following advice.

A | Acceptance of what happened

The process of recovering and making progress from a brain injury is a journey. However, that journey doesn't begin until the individual really accepts the fact that they have had a brain injury. In my daily clinical practice, I continue to encounter individuals who have had brain injuries 5, 10, 15 and even 20 years previously, who find great difficulty in coming to terms with what has happened to them and making sense of their new circumstances and moving forward. They find it difficult to accept the limitations imposed by their brain injury, failing to adapt, and consequently live or rather exist with a mindset unchanged from prior to their brain injury. They exist as relics of the past, living in a world unsuited to their present. This can be a direct consequence of the brain injury itself, if insight is affected, or it can be a consequence of the individual's way of coping.

The process of acceptance takes many parts and has many layers. The first part, however, is accepting that they have had a brain injury and that, unless their brain injury was quite mild, there will be physical, emotional and cognitive challenges as a result. Priorities, be it career or activities or relationships, cannot be the same after the injury. Similarly, a certain degree of acceptance of the need to get help and assistance from others is required.

B | Blame

Part of the process of acceptance also consists of letting go. Anger, resentment and blame are pernicious anchors that serve to hold the individual in the past and are of little help in terms of moving forward. The legal systems, both criminal and civil law, unfortunately both serve to crystallise such tendency towards blaming others. However, when there are no other individuals to blame for the brain injury, it is not uncommon – at least at a subconscious level – for the individual to blame themselves. If blame does not involve learning from past mishaps and instead consists of ruminating over those mishaps, there is little to be gained from the process. Family members can sometimes not help the situation especially if they continually remind and blame the individual for their brain injury. Similar to acceptance, at a certain point a line must be drawn in the sand and the person needs to move forward regardless of who was responsible, or otherwise, for the cause of the brain injury.

C | Clutter – of mind, possessions and environment

Earlier chapters have shown the important stabilising role of the frontal lobe in many domains, both in terms of social skills, multitasking and ultimately in executive function and organisation. Damage to the frontal lobes, therefore, is associated with a high degree of chaos. This can be seen in daily clinical practice when observing the physical appearance of an individual with a brain injury – if they lack support at home, they can come into clinic unkempt, with unruly hair and unclean clothes (such presentations aren't just limited to individuals with

frontal lobe damage, however!). The degree of chaos is far more readily apparent on home visits, when the clutter and disorganisation and
chaos of the mind is reflected in messy and disorganised rooms filled
with clothes, papers and other objects. The effect of such an untidy
environment is to exacerbate memory problems, since misplacing objects in such environments happens far easier. The presence of such
clutter and hoarding also acts as a midwife to generate more and more
clutter. The cumulative effect of all of this would be hardly any good
for the individual's own mental health and well-being.

Tidying up and organising the living environment where the individual lives, be it a room, a flat or house is absolutely vital. Inevitably
loved ones and family members have an important role in this effort,
at least in the early stages, though with time and support and encouragement, the individual can be assisted to do it themselves.

D | Daily routine

We are all creatures of habit. In ordinary daily life that habit is sustained by our jobs, our relationships and other obligations, which
mean that we get up and go to bed at regular defined times and do
various tasks at other times. Acquired brain injury presents a certain
degree of challenge to that order. Loss of job invariably (though it
should not) means loss of reasons to get up early in the morning and
consequently to go to bed at regular hours at night time. In addition,
it can reduce social contact and consequently lead to reduced financial
well-being, meaning that further constrained circumstances would
probably lead to further social isolation. In addition to being creatures
of routine, we are also creatures of meaning and the lack of meaning
and routine together can lead to a great deal of challenges in acquired
brain injury survivors.

If not done so by an occupational therapist, it is worthwhile if
the brain injury survivor and their family sit down together and create
a timetable for the week, with the timetable being as detailed as possible, trying to cover as many hours as possible during the week. Periods of rest need to be timetabled, as well as periods of when to go to

bed and when to get up in the morning. Activities need to be timetabled, including daily chores such as cleaning the house and leisure activities like going for a walk or reading a book. In the early period after discharge from hospital, it is worthwhile having the amount of activities to be somewhat limited and to gradually increase these with time. The timetable itself, however, should be displayed in a prominent position in the house and ideally on a whiteboard so that it can be modified and added to with time.

E | External control

Damage to the frontal lobes can be thought of like damaging the brakes of your car. If the handbrake on your car is not working, you do one of two things: either park it on the flat, where it is unlikely to roll, or else you might place some bricks in front and behind the wheels in the hope that the car won't move forward. In a similar way, emotional problems like anger, impulsivity and agitation can be externally managed like this.

The first way involves trying to have a settled and as stable a life as possible. This is possible and realistic for individuals who pre-brain injury lived a somewhat settled life with good family support and a stable living environment. In such cases, family members need to actively support and try and remove any potential stressors from the individual with the brain injury, particularly early on in their recuperation. They shouldn't necessarily wrap them in cotton wool but they need to be there to help deal with stresses that they know their loved one won't be able to manage.

The second means of external support is more useful in individuals who come from more chaotic environments. It is less carrots and more stick and more proactive rather than reactive. In such cases, family members need to actively identify potential sources of problems, difficulties and challenges which lead to anger, agitation or impulsive or poorly thought-out ideas on the part of the brain injury survivor. They need to put proper blocks in the way of such behaviours, either through restricting access to money, or unsavoury friends, or other

temptations such as alcohol which would worsen the individual's behaviour. It is to be hoped that with time the individual might develop
some degree of insight themselves and therefore not require the same
degree of authoritarian control. In such cases, unruly behaviour needs
to be firmly dealt with and the consequences of their actions pointed
out to them.

F | Fatigue

One of the great challenges after a brain injury is problems related to
fatigue. As already mentioned in earlier chapters, fatigue can lead to
numerous difficulties – it can worsen memory and attention and can
also lead to agitation and emotionalism. Routine and apparently mun-
dane tasks such as going in the car can be enough to make someone
more tired. The brain almost certainly repairs itself during the rest periods and sleep, particularly early on after a brain injury and therefore
regular periods of rest are essential.

G | Gym – or exercise at least!

Regular exercise is essential for all of us; in addition to helping our
physical health, it also helps our mental well-being. It will also have a
role in guarding against weight gain which can be quite common after
a brain injury, particularly if the individual is not as active as they
should be. Therefore, provision of regular exercise is essential to make
improvements. That exercise obviously does not need to be exhaus-
tive or exhausting, but it needs to be done incrementally on a graded
basis to help the individual's stamina and overall sense of well-being.
It can also serve to be an activity to get them out of the house.

H | Habit

Most of us function on autopilot throughout a lot of the day. This is
achieved through use of habits. The best example of this is early in the
morning when we automatically go through a similar series of activities in getting ourselves up, dressed, cleaned, breakfasted and out to

work. During much of the early morning, particularly if we are tired, we might not necessarily be fully aware of what we are doing so we function on autopilot, and yet it is very rare for us to leave the house without actually locking the front door or putting the alarm on. In a similar manner, even individuals with the most profound of memory problems after a brain injury can be taught to improve their overall function through habit. This is often best done by occupational therapists, but in their absence, family members can create little rituals for certain times of the day, or events such as getting up, going to bed or what to do when leaving the house. Checklists can initially be written down or written on signs and then through repetition the habits end up being learnt. Development of such habits is a good way to overcome some of the challenges associated with attentional and memory problems seen after a brain injury.

I | Insulin – the importance of regular food and water

There is little to be gained through fasting, particularly after a brain injury. One of the great challenges associated with memory problems seen after a brain injury is that the individual can forget to eat. The loss of sense of smell sometimes associated with ABI causes food to taste bland and uninteresting. The absence of the daily work routine can also mean that the habit of eating regularly at defined times becomes more chaotic. This can lead to meals being missed and the individual becomes irritable and cranky as a result of being hungry. Regular wholesome meals are therefore to be encouraged. Snack foods will give mini sugar highs and hardly improve overall behaviour. Similarly, consumption of too much caffeine can make the individual more anxious and cause insomnia. In the past, certain foods have been suggested for improving overall cognitive function, such as ginkgo biloba, B vitamins and fish oils[15]. Assuming none of such medications interact with any other medication, they are unlikely to be of huge

---

[15] Meeusen R, Decroix L. Nutritional Supplements and the Brain. *Int J Sport Nutr Exerc Metab.* 2018;28(2):200-211.

harm and may even be beneficial. However, a good balanced diet is often the best form of medication possible.

J | Job – of voluntary work

Habit and routine are great forms of rehabilitation for anyone after a brain injury. Sadly, those who have moderate to severe brain injuries frequently never return to work, which is a great pity – employment is a source of occupation and socialisation, as well as providing the individual with an income. Unfortunately, the Social Welfare system frequently is a disincentive against the individual returning to any meaningful employment. Individuals making the effort to return to work are often met with fines and a reduction in benefits by the State. However, work is a form of rehabilitation, perhaps one of the best forms of rehabilitation and if gainful employment is not practical or possible, the individual should think about voluntary work of some form to increase socialisation and self-confidence.

K | Keeping calm: temper control

Anger, agitation and outbursts are very common after a brain injury. The negative consequences of them, however, are considerable. There are many ways of trying to keep calm: avoidance of stress, taking yourself away from the situation, becoming aware of the triggers that make one annoyed, or taking a deep breath.

L | Law: the very dark side of compensation laws etc.

It is a great pity that the courts are involved in compensation and restitution of losses for injuries as a result of a brain injury. The whole process of going through the courts – be it at a civil or criminal level – is stressful for the individual and unfortunately serve to delay a sense of closure. Those going down the civil route of compensation claims end up having to run a gauntlet of seeing multiple expert medical or psychological specialists. When this gauntlet is over, they end up having to see specialists on the opposing side and answer the same questions again. Invariably, their lives become a succession of appointments at various medical rooms and solicitors' offices. The unending nature of it hardly promotes a sense of closure and good mental well-being. On top of this, individuals may end up seeing CCTV footage of the assault or accident which led to their injury; this can be very traumatic and, certainly from my clinical experience, can contribute to post-traumatic stress symptoms in their own right. Whilst in many cases avoidance of such litigation is neither possible nor practicable, the individual with the brain injury and their family should at least be aware of the challenges associated with the whole process. That said, compensation packages after a brain injury can really support the individuals further rehabilitation and quality of life.

M | Meaning – getting meaning out of things

We all need meaning in our lives. The process of happiness is not so much a destination as a journey. In an ideal world, we should derive meaning from at least four domains such as our career, family, relationships or hobbies. A well-balanced life consists of deriving a relatively equal amount of meaning out of all four areas. Whilst after a brain injury, priorities might be different, the individual, with the encouragement of their family, does need to try and continue to derive the same levels of meaning out of things and discover new activities that are joyful.

N | Notebooks and diaries

Notebooks, diaries and planners are essential after a brain injury. They can be used to fill in details on what has happened, remind the individual of what they have to do and act as an external store of information that normally the person would have been able to hold in their brain. The process of writing information into a notebook or diary is in itself both therapeutic and a way of consolidating information and assisting the person to remember. Development of computerised planners etc. means that paper does not necessarily have to be used; indeed, most mobile phones have impressive planners built into them and can be set to remind the individual to partake in various activities.

The whiteboard is uniquely useful as a reservoir of information after a brain injury and in addition to containing information on a timetable, can also remind the individual of other basic things; just the day, month, date etc. and important things they have to do on a particular day. Of all of the suggestions mentioned in this chapter, a whiteboard is one that I believe is essential and would strongly recommend purchasing.

P | Perfectionism

Conscientiousness is of great benefit in surviving and progressing forwards after a brain injury. However, perfectionism, whilst it has its positives, can also have significant negatives, particularly it if involves the individual continually berating themselves. Again, balance is required in everything in life. The ABI survivor should cut themselves slack and allow themselves to make mistakes. This can be a particular burden in individuals who have milder head injuries as they can develop a tendency to blame the brain injury for any of the 'senior moments' that we all have at all ages!

Q | Quest – the importance of ongoing goals

Life is a process of goals and trying to advance forward. It is advisable after a brain injury to have a number of simple and small goals. These can be written down in a notebook; ideally, they should be straightforward, measurable and ultimately, they need to be achievable. The process of completing goals creates its own level of satisfaction, but any goals ultimately need to be very realistic.

R | Relationships

Fundamentally, we are a social animal. One of the great tragedies of brain injuries is the effect it can have on the most sociable of individuals. It is very easy to become self-conscious and socially anxious after a brain injury, particularly if it is associated with word-finding difficulties or issues with behaviour or anger. Despite this, however, individuals after a brain injury do need to socialise. This can be with family members or friends or, in the absence of these, voluntary organisations and brain injury support groups.

S | Sex

Sex has an important role in creating feelings of intimacy and affection between couples as well as being a basic human drive. Brain injury can both diminish and increase libido. Apathy associated with frontal lobe damage, hormonal changes and side effects of medications – particularly some antidepressants – can reduce sexual interest and arousal. Frontal lobe damage can also be associated with sexual disinhibition and increased sexual demands. In any case, sexual problems are a common challenge after a brain injury and need to be discussed with the rehabilitation team or a GP. Headway have an excellent factsheet available online giving detailed information on these problems.

T | Technology

Development of computer technology, in particular integration between apps and computer programmes and other technologies, can be of vital assistance in helping the most severely brain injured. Unfortunately, social services and the NHS are frequently the last to look into such gadgets. It is therefore quite useful for the family of the individual to actively look into various technologies present for assisting and maintaining safety and quality of life for someone with a brain injury. Panic alarms and other alert buttons are available from social services. However, the last 5-10 years in particular have been associated with a huge degree of development of new technologies that frequently are unknown to the health services.

U | Understanding others

Among the general public, most will have little knowledge about brain injury. As a result, their views can often be incorrect. That ignorance can show itself in not acknowledging disability or treating those with ABI like a child. Whilst it is easy to resort to lecturing others about the effects of a brain injury, this hardly improves the overall situation and can act as a barrier to further socialisation which is so important after an ABI. Instead, sharing of gentle home truths in a diplomatic manner or giving loved ones information leaflets on brain injury can be useful in such situations.

V | Victories

In the same way that goals are important, the development of simple, achievable targets and celebrating accomplishing them is essential. It's all too easy to get preoccupied with larger goals and take for granted the minor achievements. Success in any endeavour, whether it be military campaigns or rehabilitation, is a series of minor victories. The survivor and their family members in particular need to actively celebrate the small steps gained so that confidence is present to achieve the larger steps.

W | ~~WWW~~ The dark side of the web

It goes beyond saying that the internet is a mixed bag – particularly when it comes to information on health conditions. Reputable websites such as those listed in the next chapter contain a wealth of information for brain injury survivors and their families. However, many other sites are not quite as reliable. Some will promote or attempt to sell untested and potentially dangerous treatments. Disease social forums and social media groups in particular can be of dubious benefit. Many users find a sense of comradery in discussing problems with strangers who may have had a brain injury. However, one of the problems I find associated with these forums is that they tend to focus on the negative, and the contributors can have very fixed and not necessarily objective views about treatments and therapies. In the dark early days of the rehabilitation journey a sense of hope is vital and some of these sites can crush that delicate flower.

X | X- unknown unknowns

After any brain injury the family and the survivor can have lots of questions relating to outcome and symptoms. In the absence of reassurance or a definitive answer to such queries, the brain can easily create its own catastrophic and incorrect answers. There is no such thing as a silly question, so rather than suffer in silence ask a professional.

Y | Yoga, reiki, acupuncture

Research into use of complementary medicine after brain injury is very limited. However anecdotally, many survivors report finding some of these techniques relaxing and beneficial. It's important to be aware that there are charlatans in any area and to be wary when alternative medical practitioners promise the world and charge too much. If in doubt discuss with you GP or specialist. However, some interventions such as yoga, reiki, massage, acupuncture and aromatherapy, to name a few can be very pleasant and improve general well-being, even if they don't have any proven medical benefit.

Z | Zzzz

Throughout the book the importance of sleep has been emphasised. Brain injury is quite frequently associated with insomnia and sleep problems. The following is a list of practical strategies to aid sleep.
* Try to go to bed at regular hours.
* Use the bedroom for sleeping – so no watching TV in bed, reading for hours before sleeping etc.
* Try to avoid phones and smartphones or tablet computers before bedtime.

- White noise can be very helpful, especially if you've got tinnitus. Lots of devices are available that have such noise or other relaxing sounds that can be played in the background.
- Camomile tea is great for aiding sleep. It works best to put two or even three tea bags into the cup and let it stew in the water for at least ten minutes before drinking.
- There are fantastic mindfulness and mediation programmes available on YouTube or as podcasts. If done regularly, these can help with sleep.
- Make the bedroom as sleep friendly as possible – so not too warm and not too cold, not too bright.
- Alcohol is terrible for sleep. Whilst it aids people getting to sleep, they wake up in the middle of the night and report a poor sleep.
- Be mindful that some over-the-counter medications or herbs used for sleep can have a hangover effect the next day – the antihistamines and valerian can be major offenders!

Afterword

It is very easy to think after a brain injury that you have changed as a person that everything is different and will not be the same again. However, people are strong, and usually far stronger than they realise. Fundamentally character and personality are quite stable, even after quite a catastrophic brain injury. There will still be elements of the individual that remain intact and present. In the words of Tennyson:

though much is taken much more abides and though we are not now that strength which in old days moved earth and heaven, that which we are, we are; One equal temper of heroic hearts, made weak by time and fate, but strong in will to strive, to seek, to find, and not to yield.

It is therefore important to remember, as a survivor of a brain injury, your own intrinsic value and the degree of progress that you have made and continue to make within the devastation of surviving a brain injury.

Good luck.

SOURCES OF SUPPORT

The United Kingdom

- Advice on alcohol: www.drinkaware.co.uk, www.nhs.uk/Live-well/alcohol
- Brain and Spine Foundation is a charity for individuals with brain and spine conditions 0808 808 1000 www.brainandspine.org.uk
- The Brain Tumour Charity 0808 800 0004 www.thebraintumourcharity.org.uk
- British Association of Counselling and Psychotherapy list a therapist directory to obtain psychotherapy www.bacp.org.uk
- Carers Federation 0115 9629 310 www.carersfederation.co.uk
- Carers UK 020 7378 4999 0808 808 777 adviceline@carersuk.org www.carersuk.org
- The Children's Trust is an association for children with brain injuries www.thechildrenstrust.org.uk
- The Counselling Directory 0844 8030240 www.cosrt.org.uk
- Department of Work and Pensions for information on benefits www.dwp.gov.uk
- Different Strokes is an association for young survivors of strokes 0845 130 7172 www.differentstrokes.co.uk
- Disability Horizons is an online disability lifestyle publication that offers practical advice and gives disabled people a voice www.disabilityhorizons.com
- D.V.L.A, Driver Vehicle Licence Authority. Swansea, SA99 1DL 0843 515 8104 www.gov.uk/driving-medical-conditions
- Encephalitis society is a charity that offers support and advice for individuals with encephalitis www.encephalitis.info
- Epilepsy Action 0808 800 5050 www.epilepsy.org.uk
- The Epilepsy Society 01494 601 400 www.epilepsysociaty.org.uk

- Headway is the brain injury association charity – their website is full of information on acquired brain injury with excellent downloadable booklets and local supports 0808 800 2244 helpline@headway.org.uk www.headway.org.uk
- NHS Carers Direct 0300 123 1053 www.nhs.uk/carersdirect
- Persistent vegetative state, minimally conscious or locked in syndrome support https://www.braininjuryisbig.org.uk/
- The Pituitary Foundation 0845 450 0375 www.pituitary.org.uk
- Relate – offering counselling and relationship advice 0300 100 1234 www.relate.org.uk
- Road Peace offers practical support for individuals injured in road accidents www.roadpeace.org.uk 0845 4500 355
- Stroke Association: Offers support and information on stroke. www.stroke.org.uk and Stroke helpline 0303 3033100
- The UK Council for Psychotherapy 020 7014 9955 www.psychotherapy.org.uk

Ireland

- ABI Ireland 01 280 4164 www.abiireland.ie
- Citizens Information www.citizensinformation.ie
- Headway Ireland 1800 400 478 www.headway.ie
- Irish Heart Foundation 01 6685001 https://irishheart.ie/get-support/support-groups/stroke-support-groups/
- Mental Health Ireland www.mentalhealthireland.ie
- Rehab Group https://www.rehab.ie/rehabcare/services-by-county

GLOSSARY

Acute: relating to sudden onset of symptoms

Addenbrooke's Cognitive Examination: a questionnaire that is used to determine cognitive function.

Amitriptyline: an antidepressant of the tricyclic class but used commonly at very low dose e.g. 25 mg daily to reduce pain and aid sleep

Amnesia: a deficit of memory- it may be either anterograde or retrograde.

Analgesic: pain relieving

Anhedonia: a sense of failure to enjoy things that used give pleasure, and a cardinal symptom of clinical depression

Anterior: Anatomical term relating to front

Anterograde Amnesia: impairment in the ability to form new memories

Aphasia: an impairment of language and communication that can affect the ability to understand or produce speech.

Attention: the ability of the brain to focus on one aspect of information or stimuli and not focusing on other stimuli.

Axon: the cable like extension from the nerve that carries information elsewhere.

Basal ganglia: a series of nerve cell bodies located deep within the brain that modify movement.

Beck Depression Inventory: a self-rated questionnaire used to diagnose depression in which scores greater than 33 indicate severe depression.

Blood brain barrier: a protective system within the brain that blocks substances from the blood getting into the brain.

Broca's aphasia: A language impairment that is associated with an individual understanding what others say but having difficulty in getting the words they want to say out and having a broken type of speech with word finding problems.

Central nervous system: part of the nervous system that made up of the brain and spinal cord.

Cerebellum: a part of the brain that has a role in co-ordination of movement.

Cerebrospinal fluid: a fluid that's produced deep within the brain and circulates between the ventricular system and spinal canal.

Confabulation: a deficit of memory characterised by unconsciously filling gaps in memory with fabricated facts. It is often associated with frontal lobe injury or alcoholism.

Consultant: a senior doctor usually with special training in a certain speciality.

Contusion: A region of injured tissue or skin in which blood capillaries have been ruptured; a bruise

Core training doctor (CT1-3): A junior doctor who is training within the first one to three years after foundation training. This used to be called senior houses officer.

Cortex: the top grey coloured layer of the brain that is composed of nerve cell bodies.

CT scan: an x-ray scan of the brain using a Computerised Tomography scanner

Dendrites: Arm like projections that come out of the nerve cell body of a neuron that receives information from other neurons.

Diabetes Insipidus: a disorder associated with drinking too much fluids and voiding large quantities of urine usually due to dysfunction in part of the brain that regulated fluid balance.

Diplopia: double vision

Dopamine: a neurotransmitter within the brain.

Electroencephalogram (EEG): a brain wave test that's used to diagnose epilepsy.

Executive dysfunction: higher order cognitive tasks e.g. planning, motivation, multitasking, social cues

Extradural, haematoma: a clot under the skull but on top of the protective dural layer covering the brain that leads to pressure on the underlying brain tissue

Fluency: a cognitive test that accesses the frontal lobes of the brain

Fluoxetine: an antidepressant popularly known as Prozac

Foundation Doctor: a junior doctor within the first two years of qualification as a doctor.

Frontal lobes: an area of the brain concerned with higher executive function and planning and personality

Glasgow Coma Scale (GCS): a scale for describing severity of neurological presentation and level of consciousness from 3-15, with 3 lowest score and associated with deep unconsciousness and 15 associated with normal level of alertness and good outcome.

Haemorrhagic contusions: bruising with some bleeding, in the case of the brain tissue

Hydrocephalus: increased volume of cerebrospinal fluid within the brain usually due to blockages within the ventricular system and causing damage to other brain tissue.

Intracranial pressure bolt (ICP bolt): a device used to measure the pressure inside the brain, inserted using a drill into the skull.

Intramedullary nail: an orthopaedic implant into the centre of the bone to hold it in place after a fracture.

Intubated: presence of a tube in the windpipe to assist breathing

Ischaemia: restriction of blood supply with resultant death of cells and damage due to lack of oxygen.

Korsakoff's syndrome: a condition associated with severe short-term memory problems usually due to chronic alcoholism and damage of the brain.

Lateral: anatomical term pertaining to the side

Magnetic resonance imaging: a type of imaging that used magnetic forces to form an image of the inside of the body.

Maxilla: the cheek bone

Medial: anatomical term pertaining to the centre.

Meninges: a number of protective layers of tissue that cover the brain and the inner lining of the skull. Three layers exist, the inner most Pia mater, the middle arachnoid layer and very tough our dura mater that exists just under the skull.

Mini Mental State Examination (MMSE): a very commonly used cognitive examination that is performed at the bed or deskside and that can estimate the degree of memory problems. It is scored out 30 where 30/30 is normal. However, it is a very simple type of test and doesn't really test frontal lobe function.

Motor cortex: part of the frontal lobe that controls voluntary movement.

Motor neuron: a type of nerve cell that carries information from the brain to muscles

Nerve cell body: the central part of a neuron that contains the nucleus of the cell.

Neuropsychiatrist: A medical doctor with special interest in the interface between psychiatry and neurology.

Neurotransmitter: a chemical that neurons releases in minute quantities to carry a message to another neuron, muscle or other organ.

Occipital lobe: area at the back of the brain that has a role in visual memory and use of visual information

Occupational therapist: a health professional who has special interest in helping patients redevelop new skills for daily living.

Orbit: area around the eye socket

Parietal lobe: area of the brain that Integrates sensory information

Percutaneous endoscopic gastrostomy (PEG): A tube inserted into the abdomen to feed someone when it's not possible or safe for them to eat orally.

Physiotherapist: a health professional who has special interest in treating injury with exercises, stretches and other physical techniques.

Phantom pain: a pain that appears to come from a limb that's been removed.

Posterior: an anatomical term relating to behind.

Post-traumatic amnesia: a period of confusion observed after a brain injury- associated with poorer outcome if it lasts for more than one day.

Pre-frontal cortex: part of the frontal lobe that doesn't include the motor cortex and is concerned with higher executive function.

Psychologist: a non-medical professional with training in talking therapist and formal assessment of cognition.

Radius: a bone of the forename

Rehabilitation consultant: a medical doctor with particular training in rehabilitation in rehabilitation medicine.

Reflex: an automatic unconscious movement or reaction in response to a stimulus.

Retrograde amnesia: forgetting things that happened BEFORE the trauma.

Sensory neuron: a neuron that carries sensory information from the rest of the body to the brain.

Specialty Training Doctor (ST-1-6): A more senior junior doctor who has completed core training and is now training in a particular specialty. This grade used to be called registrar or senior registrar.

Speech therapist: a health professional who has special interest in assessment of communication and swallowing difficulties and use of techniques and aids to promote communication.

Subdural haematoma: a collection of clot under the dura mater a covering of the brain. This causes brain damage due to pressure on the underlying brain tissue.

Synapse: the connection between the end of the axon in one neuron and the dendrite of another neuron.

Temporal lobe: an area of the brain concerned with memory amongst other functions

Tracheostomy: an incision in the windpipe which is made when people require assistance of machines to help them breathe.

Ventricles: cavities deep within the brain that contain cerebrospinal fluid.

Wernicke's aphasia: a language disorder associated with the individual having little understanding what others are saying and speaking fluently but not making sense.

ACKNOWLEDGEMENTS

This book has benefitted from the advice and support of many. Special thanks for reviewing the manuscripts to Dr Marc Boix, Matthew Clarke, Dr Dinesh Damodaran, Laura Davidson, Stephen Foy, Anne Jammes, Julie Jones, Dr Czarina Kirk, Dr Shagufay Mahendran, Sarah-Jane Shea, Jon Smith, and Cathy Stoneley.

CPSIA information can be obtained
at www.ICGtesting.com
Printed in the USA
LVHW031935271021
701685LV00008B/352

9 781839 190285